The Art and Science of Dermal Formulation Development

Drugs and the Pharmaceutical Sciences

A Series of Textbooks and Monographs

Series Executive Editor
James Swarbrick
PharmaceuTech, Inc. Pinehurst, North Carolina

The Art and Science of Dermal Formulation Development
Marc B. Brown and Adrian C. Williams

Pharmaceutical Inhalation Aerosol Technology, Third Edition
Anthony J. Hickey and Sandro R. da Rocha

Good Manufacturing Practices for Pharmaceuticals, Seventh Edition
Graham P. Bunn

Pharmaceutical Extrusion Technology, Second Edition
Isaac Ghebre-Sellassie, Charles E. Martin, Feng Zhang, and James Dinunzio

Biosimilar Drug Product Development
Laszlo Endrenyi, Paul Declerck, and Shein-Chung Chow

High Throughput Screening in Drug Discovery
Amancio Carnero

Generic Drug Product Development: International Regulatory Requirements for Bioequivalence, Second Edition
Isadore Kanfer and Leon Shargel

Aqueous Polymeric Coatings for Pharmaceutical Dosage Forms, Fourth Edition
Linda A. Felton

Good Design Practices for GMP Pharmaceutical Facilities, Second Edition
Terry Jacobs and Andrew A. Signore

Handbook of Bioequivalence Testing, Second Edition
Sarfaraz K. Niazi

Generic Drug Product Development: Solid Oral Dosage Forms, Second Edition
edited by Leon Shargel and Isadore Kanfer

Drug Stereochemistry: Analytical Methods and Pharmacology, Third Edition
edited by Krzysztof Jozwiak, W. J. Lough, and Irving W. Wainer

Pharmaceutical Powder Compaction Technology, Second Edition
edited by Metin Çelik

Pharmaceutical Stress Testing: Predicting Drug Degradation, Second Edition
edited by Steven W. Baertschi, Karen M. Alsante, and Robert A. Reed

Pharmaceutical Process Scale-Up, Third Edition
edited by Michael Levin

Sterile Drug Products: Formulation, Packaging, Manufacturing and Quality
Michael J. Akers

The Art and Science of Dermal Formulation Development

Marc B. Brown and Adrian C. Williams

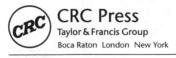

CRC Press
Taylor & Francis Group
Boca Raton London New York

CRC Press is an imprint of the
Taylor & Francis Group, an **informa** business

CRC Press
Taylor & Francis Group
6000 Broken Sound Parkway NW, Suite 300
Boca Raton, FL 33487-2742

First issued in paperback 2022

© 2019 by Taylor & Francis Group, LLC
CRC Press is an imprint of Taylor & Francis Group, an Informa business

No claim to original U.S. Government works

ISBN-13: 978-1-138-06492-8 (hbk)
ISBN-13: 978-1-03-233854-5 (pbk)
DOI: 10.1201/9780429059872

Library of Congress Cataloging-in-Publication Data

Names: Brown, Marc B., author. | Williams, A. C. (Adrian C.)
Title: The art and science of dermal formulation development / Marc B. Brown, Adrian C. Williams.
Description: Boca Raton, Florida : CRC Press, [2019] | Series: Drugs and the pharmaceutical sciences | Includes bibliographical references and index.
Identifiers: LCCN 2018051442| ISBN 9781138064928 (hardback) | ISBN 9780429059872 (ebook)
Subjects: LCSH: Transdermal medication. | Transdermal medication--Research--Methodology. | Dermatologic agents--Absorption and adsorption. | Skin--Physiology.
Classification: LCC RM151 .B76 2019 | DDC 615/.6--dc23
LC record available at https://lccn.loc.gov/2018051442

**Visit the Taylor & Francis Web site at
http://www.taylorandfrancis.com**

**and the CRC Press Web site at
http://www.crcpress.com**

We dedicate this book to our families

Marc B. Brown and Adrian C. Williams

Contents

Preface

Human skin is an attractive site for drug administration, with often-cited advantages including its accessibility, avoidance of first-pass hepatic metabolism, and the ease of cessation when adverse effects are seen. Formulations exist to deliver the active pharmaceutical ingredient to act within the skin (locally acting), at a site adjacent to the application site, such as joints or muscle beneath the skin surface (regionally acting), or at a remote site following systemic absorption (transdermal, sometimes termed "dermal", delivery). A plethora of dosage forms exist to deliver the drug molecules, from simple lotions and ointments to gels, creams, foams, and patches, and innovations such as metered sprays allow control over dosing. Topical formulations with corticosteroids, non-steroidal anti-inflammatory drugs, antiviral drugs, and anti-infective agents are widespread, and transdermal delivery systems for oestradiol, nicotine, and opioid analgesics such as fentanyl and buprenorphine are commercially successful.

The constraints on drug delivery via the skin relate to both biology and chemistry. Human skin is a remarkable self-repairing barrier that is essentially designed to keep the outsides "out" and the insides "in". Far from an inert membrane, the skin microstructure allows water loss across the tissue, but prevents ingress of microorganisms and environmental contaminants such as pollutants and toxins. As such, the skin severely restricts drug transport from the applied formulation into the body. Since the transport of most topically applied drugs is low, relatively high potency drugs are needed and, preferably, those with a relatively wide therapeutic window to mitigate the biological variability seen between skin of different patients. In chemical terms, the skin is predominantly a hydrophobic barrier, and so the physiochemical properties of the drug influence delivery – notably, the commercially successful topical products generally contain relatively lipophilic drugs such as steroids.

Simply stating that "skin is a remarkable barrier that few drugs can enter" would be a very short book, and there is much that can be done to improve and broaden the range of topically applied medicines through understanding the biological and chemical obstacles. Drug delivery can be promoted by various technological innovations, such as the use of microneedles or mild heating of the skin surface. Understanding formulation design and development, built on the theoretical principles of diffusion, can ensure optimal delivery from a topically applied product, and the ability to scale-up and quality assure a resultant formulation can help to mitigate issues arising during the manufacturing process.

This book aims to cover the above aspects, ranging from the fundamental structure and function of human skin as a barrier to drug delivery, through the underlying mathematical principles of drug permeation, to chemical and physical strategies to modulate drug delivery. The principles used to design and develop topical and transdermal formulations are then discussed along with performance testing, and finally process development and scale-up. The later chapters include case studies drawn from our experience with real-world product development.

In designing this text, we wanted to describe the whole "skin formulation" developmental pathway from early concept and principles through to product manufacture. Working in academia and industry, between us we have taught over 100 graduate (PhD) students and employed over 200 new staff to develop topical products. Our focus was to provide the initial knowledge and learning needed for these roles. Clearly, many areas in each of our chapters are the subject of more specific and detailed texts, reviews, and papers in the literature, and we have directed the interested reader to these fuller sources through the references provided. We hope that the *Art and Science of Dermal Formulation Development* provides a coherent introduction to the discipline, and that it may be a stepping-stone to further detailed study in one or more of the many diverse areas in this exciting and evolving field.

Marc B. Brown and Adrian C. Williams

Acknowledgements

We would like to express our gratitude to MedPharm and the University of Reading for allowing us the time to write this book. We would also like to acknowledge the many researchers that we have had the pleasure of working with over the last 30 years, and who have (sometimes inadvertently!) shaped the content of this text. Specifically, we would like to thank Charles Evans, James Sayer, and Cliff Fernandes for their invaluable contributions to Chapter 7, and also Yasmeen Hussain for helping design many of the figures.

> *Everybody is a genius. But if you judge a fish by its ability to climb a tree, it will live its whole life believing that it is stupid.*

Albert Einstein

About the Authors

Marc B. Brown, BSc (Hons), PhD, CChem FRSC, is the Chief Scientific Officer and Co-founder of MedPharm Ltd. He received his BSc (Hons) and PhD in Pharmaceutical Chemistry from Loughborough University. In 2006, after 14 years working as an academic at King's College London (KCL) and then as Director of Pharmaceutical Development at Hyal Pharmaceutical Corporation in Toronto, Canada, he took up a position as full-time and then part-time Chair of Pharmaceutics in the School of Pharmacy, University of Hertfordshire, where he remained until 2016. During this time, he was also awarded Honorary Professorial positions at the School of Pharmacy, University of Reading and the Institute of Pharmaceutical Science, King's College London. His research interests lie mainly in drug delivery to the skin, nail, and mucosal membranes and he has over 200 publications and 26 inventions describing his work.

In 1999 whilst at KCL, Dr Brown co-founded MedPharm Ltd, a contract research organisation specialising in the development of topical and transdermal medicines. He acts as Chief Scientific Officer of MedPharm, which employs approximately 150 people in its GMP/GLP accredited facilities in the United Kingdom and the United States. He and MedPharm have been involved in the development of 50 topical and transdermal medicines and devices that have gained regulatory approval around the world. These include two generic topical products that were approved in the European Union based on bioequivalence testing alone. These submissions utilised MedPharm's validated *in vitro* and *ex vivo* performance testing models.

Adrian C. Williams, BSc (Hons), PhD, CChem FRSC, FAPS, FHEA, is Professor of Pharmaceutics and Research Dean (Health) at the University of Reading, UK. Dr Williams started working on transdermal and topical drug delivery for his PhD in 1987, under the supervision of Professor Brian Barry at the University of Bradford. Following his doctorate, he joined the academic staff in the Bradford School of Pharmacy and continued to research varied aspects of skin structure, function, and formulation design as he progressed to Professor of Biophysical Pharmaceutics. He relocated to the School of Pharmacy at the University of Reading in 2004 and established a research group working on novel topical and transdermal formulations, as well as other areas of formulation science.

He has supervised over 50 postgraduate and postdoctoral researchers on projects funded by research councils, charities and industry. He has published over 200 articles, reviews, and book chapters which have been cited 14,000 times. Dr Williams sits on the editorial boards of the *Journal of Pharmacy and Pharmacology* and the *Journal of Pharmaceutical Sciences*, acts as a peer reviewer for national and international funding bodies and is also a member of advisory boards for international conferences and pharmaceutical companies. He is a Fellow of the Academy of Pharmaceutical Sciences and of the Royal Society of Chemistry.

Drs Brown and Williams have known each other for more than 30 years, and have worked together in supervising PhD student projects in the United Kingdom and United States.

1 Structure and Function of Human Skin

1.1 INTRODUCTION

Human skin is a remarkable barrier between the body and the environment, providing protection against ingress of allergens, chemicals, and microorganisms, regulating the loss of water and nutrients from the body and responding to mitigate the effects of ultraviolet (UV) radiation. The skin has an important role in homeostasis by regulating body temperature and blood pressure and is an important sensory organ for temperature, pressure, and pain. As the largest organ of the human body, providing around 10% of the body mass and covering an area of ~1.8 m^2 in the average person, this easily accessible tissue apparently offers ideal multiple sites to administer therapeutic agents for both local and systemic actions, but human skin is a highly efficient self-repairing barrier that has evolved to keep "the insides in and the outside out".

Skin membranes can be considered at various levels of complexity. In some mathematical treatments of transdermal drug delivery (see Chapter 2), skin can be regarded as a simple physical barrier; more complexity can be introduced by viewing the different tissue layers as multiple barriers in series. Further, drug transport through skin pores provides barriers in parallel. Degrees of complexity also exist when examining basic structures and functions of the membrane. In some extreme cases, it may be that transdermal drug delivery is limited by metabolic activity within the membrane. Alternatively, immunological responses may prevent the clinical use of a formulation that has proven to be optimal during *in vitro* studies. A further complication is introduced in clinical situations where topical delivery is intended to treat diseased skin states; here the barrier nature of the membrane may be compromised at the onset of therapy, and still further complexity is introduced if the skin barrier changes through repair during treatment.

This chapter describes the structure and function of healthy human skin, and considers some skin-related factors that can affect transdermal and topical (or "dermal") drug delivery, such as body site, the overlying skin microbiome, and age-related alterations to the membrane.

1.2 HEALTHY SKIN STRUCTURE AND FUNCTION

The anatomy of human skin is complex, but for the purpose of transdermal and topical drug delivery, we can examine its structure and function in four main layers: (1) the innermost subcutaneous fat layer (hypodermis), (2) the overlying dermis, (3) the viable epidermis, and (4) the outermost layer of the tissue (a non-viable epidermal layer) the stratum corneum. Nerves, blood, and lymphatic vessels pervade the hypodermis and dermis, and various appendages are supported in the dermis

1

and pass through to the external surface: hair follicles, eccrine glands, and apocrine glands (Figure 1.1).

It should be noted that, *in vivo*, skin is in a process of continual regeneration, is metabolically active, has immunological and histological responses to assault (as would be the case if an exogenous chemical, such as a drug, were applied to the surface), and changes due to diseased states. Due to experimental and ethical difficulties, most transdermal and topical drug delivery studies tend to use *ex vivo* (*in vitro*) skin which inherently reduces some of the above complexity – regeneration stops, immune responses cease, and metabolic activity is usually lost in these studies. Thus, with *in vitro* permeation studies, the skin effectively acts as a physical barrier to drug delivery but it should always be borne in mind that data obtained from excised skin may not translate directly to the *in vivo* situation.

1.2.1 THE SUBCUTANEOUS FAT LAYER

The subcutaneous fat layer, or hypodermis, is the deepest layer of the skin and houses major blood vessels and nerves. This layer is relatively thick in most areas of the body, typically in the order of several mm. However, there are other areas in which the subcutaneous fat layer is largely absent, such as the eyelids.

The hypodermis is composed of loose, fibrous connective tissue, which contains adipose tissue and fibroblasts. A principal role of the hypodermis is to anchor the skin to the underlying muscles, thus providing mechanical support for the skin. This layer also acts as an insulator, provides mechanical protection against physical shock and serves as a fat store of adipose tissue. The subcutaneous layer is seldom an important barrier to transdermal and topical drug delivery, since it sits below the dermis which contains a rich blood supply; for some regionally acting drugs – for

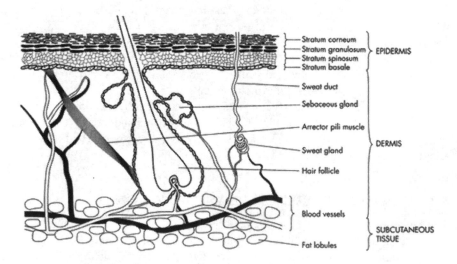

FIGURE 1.1   A diagrammatical cross-section through human skin. (From Williams, A.C., 2003. *Transdermal and Topical Drug Delivery*. London, UK: Pharmaceutical Press. With permission.)

example, those targeting joints or muscles – it is feasible that the subcutaneous layer could provide some resistance to drug delivery.

1.2.2 THE DERMIS

The dermis (or corium) is the major component of human skin and is typically 3–5 mm thick. The dermis contains fibroblasts along with adipocytes, some macrophages, and mast cells, but is also heterogeneous and two layers are evident, a lower reticular and an upper papillary layer. The reticular dermis is composed of dense irregular connective tissue, predominantly densely packed collagen fibres (providing mechanical strength) alongside elastic fibres such as elastin (for flexibility) in ground substance, an amorphous gel-like matrix that contains water, glycoproteins, and glycosaminoglycans such as hyaluronan. The reticular layer supports the blood and lymphatic vessels, nerve endings, pilosebaceous units (hair follicles and sebaceous glands), and sweat glands (eccrine and apocrine). The papillary layer overlays the reticular layer and contains more loosely arranged collagen fibres. The layer is named after the dermal papillae that interconnect the dermis with the rete ridges of the epidermis. The papillae contain terminal networks of capillaries and increase the surface area between the dermis and epidermis, which increases exchange of nutrients, waste products, and oxygen between the two layers. This also promotes transdermal drug delivery by removing permeants rapidly from the dermal–epidermal boundary. The interdigitation of the dermal papillae and epidermal rete ridges provides additional "lateral" mechanical strength to skin and the pattern of the ridges determines the patterns of fingerprints. In terms of transdermal drug delivery, the dermis is often viewed as essentially gelled water, thus providing a minimal barrier to delivery of most polar drugs, although the dermal barrier may be significant when delivering highly lipophilic molecules.

The extensive vasculature in the dermis is clearly important in regulating body temperature whilst also delivering oxygen and nutrients to the tissue and removing toxins and waste products. With regard to drug delivery, the rich blood flow, around 0.05 mL/min per mg of skin, is very efficient for the removal of molecules from the dermis to maintain the driving force for diffusion. The lymphatic system also reaches to the dermal–epidermal boundary and, whilst important in regulating interstitial pressure, facilitating immunological responses to microbial assault, and for waste removal, the lymphatic vessels may also remove permeated molecules from the dermis hence maintaining a driving force for permeation. Cross and Roberts (1993) showed that whilst dermal blood flow affected the clearance of relatively small solutes, such as lidocaine, lymphatic flow was a significant determinant for the clearance of larger molecules, such as interferon.

Three main appendages found on the surface of human skin originate in the dermis; the pilosebaceous unit, eccrine glands, and apocrine glands. In terms of transdermal drug delivery, these appendages may offer a potential route by which molecules could enter the lower layers of the skin without having to traverse the intact barrier provided by the stratum corneum. These so-called "shunt routes" may have a role to play in the early time course of the permeation process, for large polar molecules, and also in electrical enhancement of transdermal drug delivery.

However, for most permeants, the fractional area offered by these shunt routes is relatively small and so the predominant pathway for molecules to traverse the tissue remains across the bulk of the skin surface. The mechanisms by which molecules traverse human skin, including the influence of shunt route transport, are discussed in Chapter 2 (see Section 2.3).

1.2.2.1   Pilosebaceous Unit

The pilosebaceous unit consists of the hair follicle, the hair shaft, the adjoining arrector pili muscle, and the associated sebaceous gland. As the unit traverses the intact stratum corneum and epidermis, the role of the follicular pore in drug delivery has been investigated. However, as the unit is also associated with skin conditions such as acne vulgaris, folliculitis, and alopecia, the pilosebaceous unit is also a target for locally acting therapeutic agents.

The hair shaft is composed of an inner medulla overlaid with a cortex and then a cuticle. The root sheath has various layers but the outer root sheath is a keratinised layer that is continuous with the epidermis and is therefore of greatest importance with regard to drug diffusion and delivery. The hair follicle can be divided into several regions starting from the skin surface. The infundibulum is the outer part of the hair follicle and extends down to the sebaceous duct. In this area, the hair shaft is not in intimate contact with the skin and can move relatively freely. Due to the loss of epidermal differentiation, the thickness of the stratum corneum decreases deeper in the infundibulum, which results in a lesser barrier to drug diffusion compared to the stratum corneum at the skin surface.

Each hair follicle is associated with one or more sebaceous glands, outgrowths of epithelial cells, and composed of lipid-producing sebocytes lining sebaceous ducts. Non-hair bearing sites including the mouth, the eyelids, the nipples, and the genitals also have sebaceous glands. The greatest density of these glands is on the face and scalp; only the palms and soles, which also have no hair follicles, are completely devoid of sebaceous glands. The glands release lipids through holocrine secretion, and human sebum reaching the surface of the skin consists of a mixture of lipids including cholesterol, squalene, triglycerides, and free fatty acids. Sebum helps to maintain hydration and pliability of the skin's surface and provides a skin surface pH of about 5.5 which inhibits bacterial and fungal growth.

1.2.2.2   Eccrine (Sweat) Glands

The eccrine glands are simple coiled glands, 500–700 µm in diameter, located in the lower dermis. Found over most of the body surface, typically at a density of 100–200 per cm^2 of skin, eccrine glands secrete a dilute salt solution at a pH of about 5 onto the skin surface and so also confer some antimicrobial properties. Sweat secretion is stimulated by temperature-controlling determinants, such as exercise and high environmental temperature, as well as emotional stress through the autonomic (sympathetic) nervous system. Typical eccrine duct diameters are 30–40 µm.

1.2.2.3   Apocrine Glands

The apocrine glands are limited to specific areas of the skin including the axillae, nipples, and anogenital regions. The apocrine gland coil is similar in size to an eccrine gland (~800 μm in diameter), but with a significantly greater duct diameter (80–100 μm). Apocrine gland ducts secrete into the upper regions of the hair follicle, and their lipoidal and "milk" protein secretions provide nutrients for skin bacteria; bacterial decomposition of the secretions is primarily responsible for imparting the odour of sweat.

1.2.3 THE EPIDERMIS

Overlying the dermis, the epidermis is a complex multiply layered membrane which varies in thickness from around 0.06 mm on the eyelids to around 0.8 mm on the load-bearing palms and soles of the feet. The epidermis contains five histologically distinct layers, which, from the inside to the outside, are the stratum basale (also called the stratum germinativum, or simply the basal layer), stratum spinosum, stratum granulosum, stratum lucidum, and the stratum corneum (Figure 1.2). The stratum corneum, comprising anucleate (dead) cells, provides the main barrier to transdermal delivery of drugs and hence is often treated as a separate membrane by workers within the field. The term "viable epidermis" is often used to describe the underlying four distinct layers, although the viability of cells within, for example, the stratum granulosum is questionable, as the cell components degrade during differentiation.

1.2.3.1 Basement Membrane

The basement membrane delineates the dermis from the epidermis and, in essence, is the dermal–epidermal junction and anchors the epidermis to the underlying dermis. The basement membrane comprises reticular connective tissue and the basal

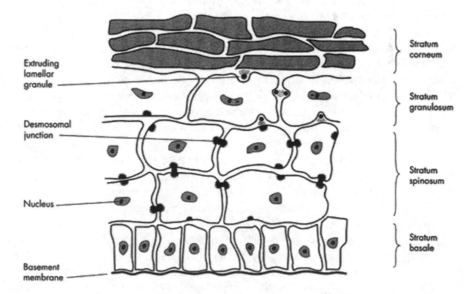

FIGURE 1.2 Diagrammatical representation of the epidermal layers and their differentiation. (From Williams, A.C., 2003. *Transdermal and Topical Drug Delivery*. London, UK: Pharmaceutical Press. With permission.)

lamina. The reticular connective tissue contains Type III collagen fibres that are synthesised by reticular cells – a specialised form of fibroblasts – and fibronectin. The basal lamina can be characterised as two layers seen by electron microscopy; an electron-dense region termed the lamina densa with reticular collagen IV fibrils and the overlaying lamina lucida, an electron-lucent region between the plasma membrane of the basal cells and the lamina densa.

In addition to maintaining epidermal–dermal adhesion, the basement membrane acts as a mechanical barrier, preventing malignant (and other) cells from migrating to the dermis. The membrane can also provide a barrier to the diffusion of large molecules from the epidermis to the dermis. The basement membrane also has a regulatory role in cell proliferation.

1.2.3.2   The Stratum Basale (Stratum Germinativum or, More Commonly, Basal Layer)

The stratum basale is a single-cell layer of columnar or cuboidal cells that are attached to the basement membrane through hemidesmosomes, using integrin to adhere the cells to the extracellular matrix, and join the overlying stratum spinosum by desmosomes. The keratinocytes of the basal layer are similar to other cells within the body in that they contain the typical organelles such as mitochondria and ribosomes and the cells are metabolically active. This layer thus contains the only epidermal keratinocytes that undergo cell division; after replication, one daughter cell remains in this layer whilst the other migrates upwards through the epidermis towards the skin surface. On average, dividing basal cells replicate once every 200 to 400 hours.

In addition to the keratinocytes, the stratum basale contains other specialised cell types. Melanocytes synthesise the pigment melanin from tyrosine. Two forms of melanin are found: eumelanin is the more common brown/black form, whereas the less common phaeomelanin is red or yellow. Melanin granules formed in the melanocytes tend to be a mixture of these two forms. Melanocytes make surface contact with adjacent keratinocytes through dendritic connections, and this allows the pigment granules to pass from the melanocytes to the keratinocytes. On facial skin, there may be up to one melanocyte for every five basal layer keratinocytes, but on less exposed surfaces, such as the trunk, this ratio may be only one melanocyte to twenty keratinocytes. Melanocyte presence appears to be inducible, with chronic exposure to light increasing the relative proportion of the pigment forming cells within the basal layer. Melanins provide an energy sink within the skin; they absorb UV radiation and are free-radical scavengers. There are equal numbers of melanocytes in a given body site in darker and lighter skin types, but darker-skinned people have more active and efficient melanocytes.

Langerhans cells are also found within the stratum basale (and in the overlying stratum spinosum as well as the papillary dermis). Langerhans cells derive from bone marrow and are recognised as the major antigen-presenting (dendritic) cells of the skin. Antigens readily bind to cell surfaces, and although Langerhans cells are not themselves efficiently phagocytic, they may present the antigens to lymphocytes in the lymph nodes. Clearly, when compared to other membranes of the body, the skin comes into contact with many potential antigens, and hence the Langerhans cells play an important role in conditions such as allergic contact dermatitis.

One other specialised cell type is found within the basal layer: the Merkel cell. These cells are found in greatest numbers around the touch sensitive sites of the body, such as the lips and fingertips. The cells are associated with nerve endings, found on the dermal side of the basement membrane, and have a role in cutaneous sensation.

1.2.3.3 The Stratum Spinosum (Spinous Layer/Prickle Cell Layer)

The stratum spinosum is found on top of the basal layer, and together these two layers are termed the Malpighian layer. This spinous layer consists of 2–6 rows of keratinocytes that change morphology from columnar to polygonal cells. Within this layer, the keratinocytes begin to differentiate and synthesise keratins that aggregate to form tonofilaments. Desmosomes connecting the cell membranes of adjacent keratinocytes are formed from condensations of the tonofilaments, and it is these desmosomes that maintain a distance of approximately 20 nm between the cells.

1.2.3.4 The Stratum Granulosum (Granular Layer)

As they pass from the stratum spinosum to the stratum granulosum, the keratinocytes continue to differentiate, synthesise keratin, and start to flatten. Only 1–3 cell layers thick, the stratum granulosum is characterised by the presence of keratohyalin granules – dense, irregular amorphous deposits that contain profilaggrin, loricrin, cysteine-rich proteins, and keratin. Profilaggrin facilitates the bundling of keratin, the major protein in corneocytes, and loricrin and cystatin-A are major compounds of the cornified cell. Importantly for topical and transdermal drug delivery, membrane-coating granules (lamellar bodies) are also synthesised, probably in the endoplasmic reticulum and Golgi apparatus, and contain the lamellar subunits arranged in parallel stacks as precursors for the intercellular lipid lamellae seen in the stratum corneum. The lamellar bodies are extruded from the cells into the intercellular spaces as the cells approach the upper layer of the stratum granulosum. At this stage, lysing enzymes are released which start to degrade viable cell components such nuclei and organelles. After this, the keratinocytes become flattened and compacted to form non-viable corneocytes.

1.2.3.5 The Stratum Lucidum

The stratum lucidum is a thin and translucent layer (hence the name) 3–5 cells thick. Here, the cell nucleus disintegrates and there is an increase in keratinisation of the cells; the cells contain eleidin, derived from keratohyalin which is then converted to keratin in the upper stratum lucidum and stratum corneum. Concomitantly, the cells undergo further morphological changes and flatten. Occasionally, droplets of an oily substance may be seen in this cell layer, probably arising from exocytosis of the lamellar bodies. The stratum lucidum tends to be seen most clearly in relatively thick skin specimens, such as from the load-bearing areas of the body (the soles of the feet and the palms). Indeed, some researchers question whether this layer is functionally distinct from the other epidermal layers, or if it is an artefact of tissue preparation. Many researchers tend to view the stratum lucidum as the lower portion of the stratum corneum and hence bracket these two layers together.

1.2.3.6   The Stratum Corneum (Horny Layer)

The stratum corneum is the final product of epidermal cell differentiation, and though it is an epidermal layer it is often viewed as a separate membrane in topical and trans-dermal drug delivery studies. The stratum corneum typically comprises only 10–15 cell layers and is 5–20 µm thick when dry, although it may swell to several times this thickness when wet. As with the viable epidermis, the stratum corneum is thickest on the palms and soles and is thinnest on the lips. This thin membrane provides the protective barrier that permits the survival of terrestrial animals without desiccation and provides the predominant obstacle to topical and transdermal drug delivery. As such, it merits deeper consideration of its structure and properties.

The stratum corneum comprises terminally differentiated keratinocytes (cor-neocytes) embedded in a multiply bilayered lipid matrix. The corneocytes are flat, polyhedral-shaped anuclear cells, approximately 40 µm in diameter and 0.5 µm thick, and contain tight bundles of intracellular keratin surrounded by a cornified cell enve-lope of covalently cross-linked proteins and covalently bound lipid. The intercellular region of the stratum corneum contains the lipids that originate primarily from the exocytosis of lamellar bodies during the terminal differentiation of keratinocytes. The upper layer of the stratum corneum is known as the stratum disjunctum and normally consists of approximately 3–5 cell layers that are actively undergoing desquamation (sloughing). The lower layer of the stratum corneum is termed the stratum compac-tum and is thicker and more densely packed than the stratum disjunctum. The stratum compactum has a higher density of corneodesmosomes than the stratum disjunctum as serine, cysteine, and aspartic proteases are excreted into the extracellular spaces to break the desmosomes for desquamation. It typically takes 14 days for a daughter cell from the stratum basale to differentiate into a stratum corneum cell, and the stratum corneum cells are typically retained for a further 14 days prior to shedding.

The stratum corneum has been represented as a "bricks and mortar" model in which the corneocytes are embedded in a mortar of lipid bilayers (Figure 1.3). However, it should be borne in mind that the corneocytes are polygonal, elongated, and relatively flat, and that the lipid mortar is a series of multiple lipid bilayers. The barrier nature of the stratum corneum depends critically on its unique constituents; the corneocyte keratin is predominantly α-keratin (around 70%), a fibrous struc-tural protein that forms coiled coils with disulphide bonds between two helices. This provides structural stability and some degree of deformation to stretch and absorb impact. In addition, β-keratin (approximately 10%) is found in pleated sheets and provides additional rigidity, whilst the proteinaceous cell envelope (around 5%) is highly insoluble and very resistant to chemical attack. The cell envelope also has a key role in structuring and ordering the intercellular lipid lamellae of the stratum corneum; the corneocyte is bound to lipids through glutamate moieties of the protein envelope. The lipid envelope thus provides an anchor to the keratinocyte and links the proteinaceous domains of the keratinocytes to the intercellular lipid domains.

Human stratum corneum contains a unique mixture of lipids and, for most perme-ants, the continuous multiply bilayered lipid component of the stratum corneum is key in

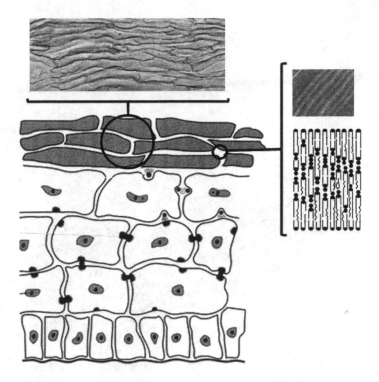

FIGURE 1.3 Illustration and electron micrographs of the "bricks and mortar" structure of human stratum corneum.

regulating drug flux through the tissue (see Chapter 2). The crucial role of the SC lipids in the barrier function has been demonstrated following their removal by solvent extraction, which leads to increased transepidermal water loss and enhanced skin permeability.

Unlike other membranes in the human body, the stratum corneum lipid bilayers are not formed from phospholipids. The lamellar bodies of the stratum granulosum contain glucosylceramides, sphingomyelin, and phospholipids; these precursors are enzymatically processed into ceramides and free fatty acids by hydrolytic enzymes, and, together with cholesterol, form the multiple lipid bilayers of the stratum corneum. The free fatty acids essentially contain a single carbon chain, whereas the ceramides have two carbon chains; in human stratum corneum, the free fatty acids, ceramides, and cholesterol are found in near-equimolar ratios.

The SC intercellular lipid lamellae are highly structured both in terms of their lamella and their lateral packing. In terms of their lamella, two co-existing phases are seen; a short periodicity phase (with a repeat distance of ~6.4 nm between lipid head groups) and a long periodicity phase (with repeat distance of ~13.4 nm). Three states of lateral lipid organisation have been identified; a highly ordered densely packed orthorhombic phase which is crystalline and exhibits low permeability to drug molecules, an ordered less densely packed, gel-like, more permeable hexagonal phase and a disordered, highly permeable liquid phase. Within the SC, the orthorhombic packing is generally accepted to be the dominant phase in healthy skin (Figure 1.4).

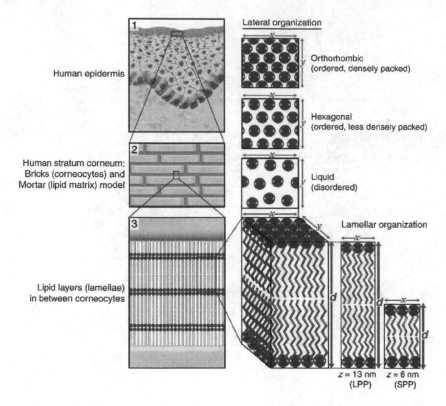

FIGURE 1.4   Lateral and lamellar packing of stratum corneum lipids. (From van Smeden, J., Janssens, M., Gooris, G.S., and Bouwstra, J.A., 2014. The important role of stratum corneum lipids for the cutaneous barrier function. *Biochim. Biophys. Acta (BBA) Mol. Cell Biol. Lipids* 1841: 295–313. With permission.)

Recent advances in analytical methodologies have revealed remarkable variety in free fatty acid and ceramide composition in human stratum corneum, and indicates that this varies with body site. The free fatty acids are largely saturated (~60%) but significant proportions of hydroxy- (~20%) and mono-unsaturated fatty acids (~20%) are also found. In terms of chain length, C18, C24, and C26 are most predominant, but chain lengths from C12 to C36 have also been reported.

Greater complexity is seen in the ceramide composition of the stratum corneum. In essence, ceramides comprise a fatty acid attached to a sphingoid base. Four sphingoid bases have been described: sphingosine, dihydrosphingosine, phytosphingosine, and 6-hydroxy-4-sphingenine, each with varying carbon chain lengths between C14 and C28. The fatty acids attached to the sphingoid base also vary, with acyl chains ranging from C14 to C32. The fatty acids may be non-hydroxylated, α-hydroxy or ω-hydroxy esterified. With four sphingoid bases and three different classes of fatty chain, 12 ceramide sub-classes have been described, though with variability in chain length composition within each sub-class. Phytosphingosine with non-hydroxy fatty acid chains is the most abundant sub-class (around 25% of the total ceramide content) and ultra-long ceramides (>C28) comprise around 10% of the total (Figure 1.5).

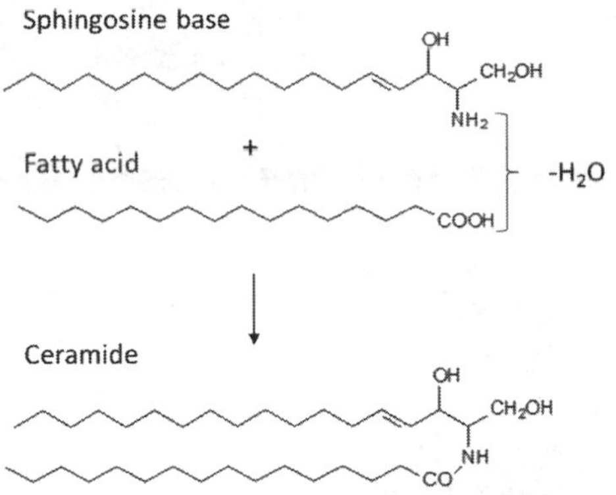

FIGURE 1.5 General scheme for the structure of stratum corneum ceramides with a sphingoid base and fatty acid chain.

It should be noted that the stratum corneum lipid composition and organisation can be significantly affected in diseased states such as psoriasis, atopic dermatitis, and lamellar ichthyosis. This may result from changes in proliferation and differentiation of keratinocytes and/or the effects of inflammation on lipid biosynthesis. For example, in atopic dermatitis, an increase in short chain lipids and unsaturated fatty acids is seen. The consequence of these biosynthetic differences in diseases states is to generally reduce the barrier function of the intercellular lipid domains compared to normal healthy human skin.

In addition to the keratinocytes and lipid lamellae, water plays a key role in maintaining stratum corneum barrier integrity since it is a plasticiser and thus prevents the stratum corneum from cracking due to mechanical assault. The outer stratum disjunctum contains approximately 15% (w/w) water, whereas the lower regions of the stratum corneum typically contain ~30% (w/w) water; both values are lower than the underlying viable dermis (70% by weight) and hence a water gradient exists through the skin. Water also mediates the activity of some hydrolytic enzymes within the stratum corneum, since environmental humidity affects the activities of enzymes involved in the desquamation process. Additionally, keratinocyte water activity regulates enzymes involved in the generation of Natural Moisturising Factor (NMF).

Natural Moisturising Factor is a highly efficient humectant synthesised, and hence located, within the stratum corneum. A proteolytic product from filaggrin (**fil**ament **aggr**egating prote**in**), NMF is essentially a mixture of free amino acids, amino acid derivatives, and salts; serine, glycine, pyrrolidone carboxylic acid, citrulline, alanine, and histidine are the major components, with lesser amounts of arginine, ornithine, urocanic acid, and proline. This hygroscopic mixture retains moisture within the stratum corneum and helps to maintain suppleness. Ten to twelve filaggrin units are post-translationally hydrolysed from the precursor profilaggrin. Mutations to the filaggrin gene have been associated with various dry skin conditions and eczema, illustrating the importance of NMF in maintaining the stratum corneum water balance.

On the surface of the stratum corneum, the acid mantle is a thin protective film comprised of sebum, corneocyte debris, and remnant material from sweat. Sebum is the principal component and is largely triglycerides, wax esters and squalene, though the composition and secretion of these differ by anatomical region. The mantle provides an acidic surface to the stratum corneum, in the region of pH 5 in comparison to the viable epidermis pH of around 7.4. The acid mantle thus provides a non-specific defence mechanism against the ingress of pathogenic organisms; if adapted to the slightly acid surface pH, once within the more alkaline environment of the viable epidermis, the pathogens are poorly adapted to survive. In terms of drug delivery, it is theoretically feasible that the acid mantle could affect the ionisation of applied drugs or that its lipids could provide an additional barrier to drug permeation, but in practice this very thin layer is seldom regarded as a significant obstacle to drug delivery.

1.2.4 EPIDERMAL ENZYME SYSTEMS

From the above, it is apparent that human skin contains many enzymes – for example, stratum corneum tryptic and chemotryptic proteases – that are required for specific purposes such as desquamation. In addition, the epidermis contains many drug-metabolising enzymes. Histochemical and immunohistochemical methodologies suggest that the majority of these are localised in the viable epidermis, sebaceous glands, and hair follicles. Although present at relatively small quantities in comparison to the liver, they do allow metabolic activity that can effectively reduce the bioavailability of topically applied medicaments; a common misconception is that the skin is an "inert" tissue. Indeed, most Phase 1 (e.g., oxidation, reduction, hydrolysis) and Phase 2 (e.g., methylation, glucuronidation) reactions can occur within the skin, though these tend to be at <10% of the specific activities found in the liver. However, esterases tend to have relatively high activities within skin and, considering that there is a large skin surface area, metabolism of some drugs can be significant in some cases. This metabolic activity can be exploited in the delivery of prodrugs such as steroid esters with the increased lipophilicity afforded by an aliphatic chain improving drug uptake into the tissue where esterases can liberate the free drug within the skin. Microorganisms present on the skin surface, such as *Staphylococcus epidermidis* may also metabolise topically applied drugs.

1.3 PHYSIOLOGICAL FACTORS AFFECTING TRANSDERMAL AND TOPICAL DRUG DELIVERY

There are a number of physiological factors that affect the structure of healthy human skin, some of which may consequently influence topical and transdermal drug delivery.

1.3.1 GENDER

A number of differences between male and female skin have been reported (Giacomoni et al., 2009). Many of these discrepancies are under hormonal control and arise from the sex steroid differences between males and females. On androgenic hormone stimulation, the sebaceous glands increase in both size and secretory activity; Caucasian men have been reported to have larger pores and greater sebum production ($3 \ \mu g/cm^2$) than women ($0.7 \ \mu g/cm^2$).

Subjected to physical exercise, males tend to sweat at a greater rate (~800 mL/h) than females (~450 mL/h). Since sweat and sebum affect skin surface pH, minor variations have been reported between the genders. Measuring the pH (hydrogen ion activity) of skin is inherently problematic and tends to use washings from the skin surface or from skin where the stratum corneum has been stripped. Under these conditions, the skin surface pH of males was reported to be 5.8 whereas in females it was 5.5 (Ehlers et al., 2001), and epidermal pH (stratum corneum removed) from the interstitial fluid was 4.6 in males and 5.6 in females (Jacobi et al., 2005).

Gender differences in gross skin thickness (dermis and epidermis) have also been reported with male skin thicker than female at all ages. Female skin has been reported to be approximately 10% thinner post-menopause and ovarectomy is associated with thinning of the skin, whereas oestrogen therapy thickens skin in females. Skin thickness generally decreases with age; this is generally associated with loss of collagen rather than alterations to the stratum corneum barrier.

Whilst these gender-related differences, particularly in pore size and surface pH could theoretically affect topical and transdermal drug delivery, in practice, most studies report no differences in permeability between male and female skin. Similarly, transepidermal water loss (TEWL) is invariant between the sexes.

1.3.2 SKIN AGE

Changes to human skin on ageing have been extensively studied, both for drug delivery and for the use of pharmaceutical and cosmetic preparations. It is widely recognised that skin undergoes structural changes on ageing, with both the dermis and epidermis thinning; levels of collagen and elastin decline with age. Blood flow (dermal clearance of molecules traversing the tissue) tends to decrease with age and this could, in theory, reduce transdermal drug flux. However, for the majority of permeants, dermal clearance tends not to be the rate-limiting factor in transdermal therapy. Further, adhesion between corneocytes reduces and the number of melanocytes and Langerhans cells falls over time. In addition to these intrinsic biological changes, lifetime environmental exposure to solar radiation and exogenous chemicals (including soaps, cosmetics, or pharmaceutical active ingredients) can also affect the structure and barrier performance of skin.

Some age-related changes to the stratum corneum have been reported, in particular to its intracellular lipid composition (Rogers et al., 1996). There are significant decreases in the levels of ceramides, as well as cholesterol and fatty acids, on ageing; as an interesting aside, there were also seasonal variations – lower levels in winter when compared to summer – in the stratum corneum lipid compositions. However, the significance of these alterations on the stratum corneum barrier function and for topical and transdermal drug delivery remains uncertain. Transepidermal water loss declines with age, but most permeation studies report no significant difference in skin permeability with age, especially for molecules such as oestradiol and testosterone. With an age-related decrease in Natural Moisturising Factor reducing the water content of elderly skin, it is feasible that permeation of polar molecules such as benzoic acid or caffeine could be reduced with age (Roskos et al., 1989) but the inherent variability of the tissue and the application of either water-based or occlusive formulations is likely to either obscure or mitigate these changes.

Whilst the ageing effects of normal mature skin on drug delivery are minimal, there are important morphological and hence permeability differences between mature skin and that of a newborn or neonate (pre-term infant). Skin development within the embryo begins approximately a week after conception with the formation of a single epithelial layer. This differentiates into epidermal and dermal tissue, but at (normal mature) birth, the dermis is only around 60% of its adult thickness; maturity of the dermis takes 3–5 months after birth. Within the embryo, a temporary outer skin layer called the periderm forms towards the end of the first month, which then thins towards the end of the second trimester concomitant with the appearance of a stratum corneum. However, the stratum corneum of the fetus is somewhat different to that of an adult, and it remains as a very thin membrane of only a few cell layers thick until shortly before birth. Thus, the immature fetus has an impaired skin barrier, but advances in medical care are allowing neonates to survive from as early as 26 weeks.

There are concerns associated with the imperfect skin barrier of the neonate; the surface area to body weight ratio may be four times that in an adult, causing difficulties with thermoregulation, transepidermal water loss, infection, and absorption of exogenous chemicals. However, the reduction in the skin barrier properties can be advantageous for delivery of drugs to the neonate; typically, antibiotics, analgesics, and cardiovascular and respiratory drugs need to be administered in a controlled manner. Oral therapy is problematic, and intravenous administration, though the norm, is difficult. Transdermal delivery has been successfully used to deliver clinical levels of caffeine and theophylline to neonates. However, it is not possible to provide a general transdermal formulation for drug delivery across neonatal skin; neonates vary in gestation time (and hence in the degree of stratum corneum immaturity, and consequently in the permeability of the tissue) and the neonatal stratum corneum matures post-delivery.

1.3.3 BODY SITE

It is readily apparent that skin structure varies to some degree over the human body; clearly the stratum corneum is thicker on the palms of the hands and soles of the feet (i.e., the load-bearing areas of the body) than on the lips or eyelids. However, the relative permeability of different skin sites is not simply a function of stratum corneum thickness, since different permeants exhibit varied rank orders through different skin sites. Wester and Maibach (1999), in reviewing regional (site to site) variations in permeability, showed that variations in drug absorption can be seen for sites with a similar thickness of stratum corneum, and that some areas with different stratum corneum thickness provide similar levels of drug absorption. In addition to stratum corneum thickness, the corneocyte surface area varies, and follicular density and the volume of pores differs from site to site. Regional variations in cutaneous blood flow and transepidermal water loss have also been reported.

Though site-to-site variation in permeability is clearly multi-factoral and complex, there are some general trends shown in the numerous literature reports on the subject. Almost 50 years ago, Feldman and Maibach (1970) described regional variation of hydrocortisone skin permeation with greatest absorption across scrotal skin, some 42 times greater than that seen with application to the ventral forearm, and the lowest absorption was observed through the heel. It is apparent that genital tissue usually provides the most permeable site for transdermal drug delivery. The skin of the head and neck is also relatively permeable compared to other sites of the body, such as the arms and legs. Intermediate permeabilities for most drugs are found on the trunk of the body. Thus, a generalised rank order of site permeabilities is:

$$\text{genitals} > \text{head and neck} > \text{trunk} > \text{arm} > \text{leg}$$

Thus there is a clear scientific rationale for selecting the application site based on permeability; scrotal tissue is the most permeable and hence offers the greatest prospect of drug delivery to clinical levels. Indeed, transdermal delivery of testosterone is highly effective through scrotal skin, but delivering drugs through scrotal tissue is restricted to around half of the population. For convenience, the trunk, upper arm, or upper leg is often selected as a site of intermediate relative permeability for application of patches, since these tend to be relatively hair free areas for ease of removal and flex less during exercise than other regions, and hence improve patient compliance. Alternatively, the relatively high permeability of skin on the head is used for scopolamine delivery; patches are applied to the postauricular (behind the ear) region where skin permeability is relatively high.

The regional variations in transdermal drug absorption should be contextualised with respect to variation found for the same site between different individuals (Southwell et al., 1984). There is, as would be expected for a biological membrane, considerable variation in permeation across a given body site (e.g., the trunk) of an individual (up to around 30% *in vitro*) and also considerable variation between the same body site on different individuals (up to around 40% *in vitro*). Whilst the degree of variability is likely to be lower *in vivo* and is permeant-dependent, this variability can exceed that resulting from regional differences if using tissue from, for example, the arm and the leg where the regional factor is small.

1.3.4 RACE

Historically, few reports describe differences in the stratum corneum barrier function or drug delivery into or through skin from different ethnic backgrounds. Studies showed marginal or no differences in transepidermal water loss or in the delivery of benzoic acid, nicotine, and aspirin between African, Asian, and European skin (Berardesca and Maibach, 1990; Lotte et al., 1993).

However, there are significant differences in the stratum corneum water content between races (Berardesca et al., 1991) and it would be anticipated that these differences in hydration would be apparent through differences in drug absorption. More recently, Muizzuddin et al. (2010) reported on structural and functional differences of African American, Caucasian, and East Asian skin. Baseline transepidermal water loss (*in vivo*) was lower in the African American skin (5.6 ± 2.2 g.h/m^2) than for East Asians (7.8 ± 3.1 g.h/m^2) and highest for Caucasians (10.2 ± 2.4 g.h/m^2). As a measure of ceramide content, the amounts of the C18 phytosphingosine-based ceramides also varied; Caucasian and East Asian volunteers had similar levels of the ceramide in their stratum corneum (1.18 ± 0.46 and 1.14 ± 0.51 µg/mg respectively), with significantly lower levels in the African American skin (0.74 ± 0.25 µg/mg). However, African American skin has a greater number of keratinocyte layers, with high cellular cohesion within the stratum corneum, and this increase in stratum corneum thickness and its maturation resulted in a "strong" stratum corneum barrier, whereas the stratum corneum barrier was weakest in the skin of the East Asian panel. The results may partially explain the differences in skin sensitivity or skin reactivity that have been reported to be higher in Asian skin.

In light of the regional, intra- and inter-site variability described above, variations in stratum corneum structure between ethnic groups appears to be of marginal importance for topical and transdermal drug delivery.

1.3.5 OTHER FACTORS

The level of hydration of the stratum corneum can have a significant effect on drug permeation through the tissue. As described above, Natural Moisturising Factor declines with age, which can alter the pliability of the skin, as well as potentially reducing delivery of polar molecules. Null mutations of the filaggrin gene reduce the levels of NMF in the tissue and are related to dry skin conditions, which can also affect topical and transdermal drug delivery. It is well-established that increasing stratum corneum hydration tends to increase transdermal delivery of most drugs. The basis for hydration elevating flux of both lipophilic and hydrophilic permeants has been extensively studied; increasing water activity in the stratum corneum causes the keratinocytes to swell which would intuitively increase partitioning and hence delivery of hydrophilic drugs (Van Hal et al., 1996). Some pooling of excess water may occur in the intracellular lipid lamella and separation and compaction of the lipid bilayers forming cisternae was reported from high-resolution cryo-scanning electron microscopy (Tan et al., 2010). Occlusive dressings and patches are highly effective strategies to increase transdermal drug delivery, since they create elevated hydration of the stratum corneum by preventing (or markedly reducing) transepidermal water loss. However, inter-individual variations in the level of stratum corneum hydration on occlusion may lead to variable drug absorption, and prolonged occlusion of the skin can lead to irritation and, potentially, microbial growth beneath an occlusive patch or dressing.

Since diffusion through the stratum corneum is a passive process, increasing the temperature clearly increases the permeant diffusion coefficient (at a fixed concentration gradient: see Chapter 2). The human body maintains a temperature gradient across the skin from around 37°C inside to around 32°C at the outer surface. Moderate heating of the skin, for example with heating pads of self-heating patches (Chapter 4, Section 4.8), increases drug flux predominantly by increasing drug release from a formulation and increasing drug diffusivity within the stratum corneum (Wood et al., 2012). In addition, temperature affects the vasculature and sweat production, which can also influence drug delivery. Greatly elevating the skin temperature (>55°C) can induce structural alterations to the stratum corneum lipids and can denature proteins, and these modifications can radically increase diffusion through the tissue. In general, minor variations in skin or environmental temperatures tend to have minimal effects on transdermal or topical drug delivery.

1.4 SKIN MICROBIOME

It has recently been estimated that the human body contains approximately 30 trillion (3×10^{12}) cells, and 37 trillion bacteria (Sender et al., 2016). Research into the gut microbiome is relatively mature, and has shown associations between the gut microbiota and, amongst others, irritable bowel disease, cardiovascular disease, and impacts on signalling via the gut–brain axis. Through technological advances allowing rapid gene sequencing, the skin microbiome is now the subject of interest, as recently reviewed by Byrd et al. (2018).

Skin is populated with bacteria (and yeasts, fungi, and viruses) at birth, the initial composition of which is dependent on the mode of delivery (vaginal or Caesarian). The immature immune system allows colonisation of the skin surface without stimulating inflammatory responses and thus the skin microbiota educates the innate and adaptive arms of the cutaneous immune system. Once mature, different microorganisms elicit distinct effects on the immune system to maintain commensal bacteria and eliminate possible pathogens. There is thus some "communication" between the skin microbiota, epithelial cells, and innate and adaptive immune systems. Keratinocytes sense microorganisms, especially their pathogen-associated molecular patterns (PAMPs), through pattern recognition receptors (PRRs). Binding of PAMPs to PRRs triggers innate immune responses, resulting in the secretion of antimicrobial peptides that can rapidly kill and inactivate fungi, bacteria, and parasites.

In contrast to the gut microbiome which stabilises at around three years of age, the skin microbiome alters during puberty when sebum production increases. This facilitates the growth of more "lipophilic" bacteria such as *Propionibacterium* spp. and fungi such as *Malassezia* spp. These age-related changes in the skin microbiota may correlate with the prevalence of some skin disorders such as acne.

Biotransformations of topically applied drugs by endogenous skin enzymes were described above (Section 1.2.4). Given the bacterial burden on the skin surface, then it is feasible that the skin microbiome could also influence sustained transdermal delivery of, in particular, biological-active ingredients such as peptides or proteins, and for some "natural" materials such as glucosamine (Tekko et al., 2006). Skin microbiota varies from site to site with greater diversity of bacterial species seen on the arm than on the scalp or armpit (Perez-Perez et al., 2016). Samples from six ethnic groups – Caucasian-American (U.S.-born, of European ancestry), African American, and men born in Africa (African Continental), East Asia, Latin America, or South Asia – all showed significant differences in bacterial composition at the different sites. For most topically applied drugs, the influence of the skin microbiome on drug transformations is likely to be marginal in the context of site-to-site and intra-patient variability.

1.5 DAMAGED SKIN

The above considered intact healthy skin with a fully developed and functioning stratum corneum. The stratum corneum barrier can be compromised by exposure to radiation, irritant chemicals, and allergens, as well as through trauma. Damage to the skin is often accompanied by an inflammatory response, which can reduce the stratum corneum barrier and increase topical and transdermal drug delivery. It is readily apparent that skin damage and disorders will affect the nature of the skin barrier and hence will influence topical and transdermal drug delivery. Indeed, many formulations are applied topically to damaged and diseased skin, such as in psoriasis or atopic dermatitis. Clearly, for many skin disorders where the barrier function is compromised, as treatment progresses the condition will improve, in other words, the barrier function of the tissue may be restored to that approaching uninvolved tissue and consequently, as the disorder improves, drug delivery decreases. Further complication is introduced when topical formulations are applied to treat skin disorders which may themselves affect the stratum corneum barrier. Topical corticosteroids tend to reduce the stratum corneum thickness and topical retinoids enhance desquamation, thus reducing the stratum corneum thickness and barrier function.

There are hundreds of skin conditions that affect humans, ranging from acne and atopic dermatitis to infections, cancers, psoriasis, and vitiligo. The American Academy of Dermatology, drawing on data from health care claims, recently reported that one in every four Americans saw a clinician for a skin condition in 2013; over 24 million visits were for non-cancerous skin growths, 3 million for atopic dermatitis, and 1.6 million visits were for psoriasis. According to the British Skin Foundation, 60% of British people currently suffer from or have suffered from a skin disease at some point during their lifetime.

For example, acne is estimated to affect 9.4% of the global population (Tan and Bhate, 2015), most commonly in post-pubescent teens, though it also persists into adulthood. Simplistically, acne occurs when hair follicles and their associated sebaceous gland are obstructed with sebum and/or dead keratinocytes. This blockage appears as a "blackhead". When the follicular opening contains the normal skin anaerobe, *Propionibacterium acnes*, lipases from the bacterium can metabolise sebum triglycerides into free fatty acids, which irritate the follicular wall and form pustules, or "whiteheads", often with inflammation of the surrounding tissue. Since sebum production is under androgenic control, hormonal changes through puberty tend to initiate acne, and genome-wide association studies suggest that androgen metabolism regulating genes can increase susceptibility to acne; genetic variation in *P. acnes* may also be a factor. There is some evidence that the stratum corneum barrier is inherently impaired in patients with acne vulgaris (Yamamoto et al., 1995), with decreased levels of free sphingosine and ceramides in the stratum corneum of acne-prone individuals. These changes correlated with an increase in transepidermal water loss and decreased SC hydration (measured by conductance) for patients with moderate acne when compared to those with a mild version of the condition.

Loss-of-function mutations in the FLG gene, coding for filaggrin, is associated with reduced levels of Natural Moisturising Factor and an impaired stratum corneum barrier in those with atopic dermatitis (AD). Transepidermal water loss from both involved and non-involved sites is elevated in AD suffers compared to that from normal healthy subjects; delivery of theophylline through AD skin was also elevated with mean fluxes of 12.5, 9.8, and 4.9 µg/cm^2/h through lesional and non-lesional AD skin and healthy normal skin respectively (Yoshiike et al., 1995). Similarly, transepidermal water loss is elevated in psoriatic skin lesions. However, whilst the barrier impairment may increase topical drug delivery, depending on disease severity, then the presence of thickened hyperkeratotic plaques may in fact decrease the flux of some drugs and uptake of active pharmaceutical ingredients into the plaques may be greater than uptake into normal stratum corneum (Anigbogu et al., 1996).

As with most medical specialisms, dermatology is rapidly developing in terms of understanding the genetic associations with diseases, the consequences of gene mutations on protein expression (proteomics), and small molecule signalling and metabolism (metabolomics). Through these advances, molecular disease markers are supporting clinical decision-making and differentiation of disease sub-types, and personalised and precision medicines promise targeted therapies tailored to an individual patient's pathophysiology. Consequently, emergent classes of active pharmaceutical ingredients are growing from small organic molecules to biomacromolecules such as monoclonal antibodies. Delivery of these macromolecules through intact skin is problematic, but given their potency and that the skin barrier is often compromised in diseased states, opportunities exist to design topically applied formulations for these agents.

REFERENCES

Anigbogu, A.N.C., Williams, A.C., and Barry, B.W. (1996). Permeation characteristics of 8-methoxypsoralen through human skin; relevance to clinical treatment. *J. Pharm. Pharmacol.* 48: 357–366.

Berardesca, E. and Maibach, H.I. (1990). Racial differences in pharmacodynamic response to nicotinates in vivo in human skin: black and white. *Acta Derm. Venereol.* 70: 63–66.

Berardesca, E., de Rigal, J., Leveque, J.L., and Maibach, H.I. (1991). In vivo biophysical characterisation of skin physiological differences in races. *Dermatologica* 182: 89–93.

Byrd, A.L., Belkaid, Y., and Segre, J.A. (2018). The human skin microbiome. *Nat. Rev. Microbiol.* 16: 143–155.

Cross, S.E. and Roberts, M.S. (1993). Subcutaneous absorption kinetics of interferon and other solutes. *J. Pharm. Pharmacol.* 45: 606–609.

Ehlers, C., Ivens, U.I., Møller, M.L., Senderowitz, T., and Serup, J. (2001). Females have lower skin surface pH than men. *Skin Res. Technol.* 7: 90–94.

Feldman, R. and Maibach, H.I. (1970). Absorption of some organic compounds through the skin in man. *J. Invest. Dermatol.* 54: 399–404.

Giacomoni, P.U., Mammone, T., and Teri M. (2009). Gender-linked differences in human skin. *J. Dermatol. Sci.* 55: 144–149.

Griffiths, C., Barker, J., Bleiker, T., Chalmers, R., and Creamer, D. (Eds.) (2016). *Rook's Textbook of Dermatology*, 9th edn. Chichester, U.K.: John Wiley and Sons.

Jacobi, U., Gautier, J., Sterry, W., and Ladermann, J. (2005). Gender-related differences in the physiology of the *Stratum Corneum*. *Dermatology* 211: 312–317.

Lotte, C., Wester, R.C., Rougier, A., and Maibach, H.I. (1993). Racial differences in the in vivo percutaneous absorption of some organic compounds: a comparison between black, Caucasian and Asian subjects. *Arch. Dermatol. Res.* 284: 456–459.

Muizzuddin, N., Hellmans, L., Overloop, L.V., Corsjens, H., Declerq, L., and Maes, D. (2010). Structural and functional differences in barrier properties of African American, Caucasian and East Asian skin. *J. Dermatol. Sci.* 59: 123–128.

Perez-Perez, G.I., Gao, Z., Jourdain, R., Ramirez, J., Gany, F., Clavaud, C., Demaude, J., Breton, L., and Blaser, M.J. (2016). Body site is a more determinant factor than human population diversity in the healthy skin microbiome. *PLoS One* 11(4): e0151990. doi:10.1371/journal.pone.0151990

Rogers, J., Harding, C., Mayo, A., Banks, J., and Rawlings, A. (1996). Stratum corneum lipids: the effect of ageing and the seasons. *Arch. Dermatol. Res.* 288: 765–770.

Roskos, K.V., Maibach, H.I., and Guy, R.H. (1989). The effect of aging on percutaneous absorption in man. *J. Pharmacokinet. Biopharm.* 17: 617–630.

Sender, R., Fuchs, S. and Milo, R. (2016). Revised estimates for the number of human and bacteria cells in the body. *PLoS Biol.* 14: e1002533.

Southwell, D., Barry, B.W., and Woodford, R. (1984). Variations in permeability of human skin within and between specimens. *Int. J. Pharm.* 18: 299–309.

Tan, G., Xu, P., Lawson, L.B., He, J., Freytag, L.C., Clements, J.D., and John, V.T. (2010). Hydration effects on skin microstructure as probed by high-resolution cryo-scanning electron microscopy and mechanistic implications to enhanced transcutaneous delivery of biomacromolecules. *J. Pharm. Sci.* 99: 730–740.

Tan, J.K.L. and Bhate, K. (2015). A global perspective on the epidemiology of acne. *Br. J. Dermatol.* 172: 3–12.

Tekko, I.A., Bonner, M.C., Williams, A.C. (2006). An optimised reverse-phase high performance liquid chromatographic method for evaluating percutaneous absorption of glucosamine hydrochloride. *J. Pharm. Biomed. Anal.* 41: 385–392.

Van Hal, D.A., Jeremiasse, E., Junginger, H.E., Spies, F., and Bouwstra, J.A. (1996). Structure of fully hydrated human stratum corneum: a freeze fracture electron microscopy study. *J. Invest. Dermatol.* 106: 89–95.

van Smeden, J., Janssens, M., Gooris, G.S., and Bouwstra, J.A. (2014). The important role of stratum corneum lipids for the cutaneous barrier function. *Biochim. Biophys. Acta (BBA) Mol. Cell Biol. Lipids* 1841: 295–313.

Wester, R.C. and Maibach, H.I. (1999). Regional variation in percutaneous absorption. In: Bronaugh, R.L. and Maibach, H.I. (Eds.), *Percutaneous Absorption; Drugs – Cosmetics – Mechanisms – Methodology*, 3rd edn. New York: Marcel Dekker Inc., pp. 107–116.

Williams, A.C. (2003). *Transdermal and Topical Drug Delivery*. London, UK: Pharmaceutical Press.

Wood, D.G., Brown, M.B., and Jones, S.A. (2012). Understanding heat facilitated drug transport across human epidermis. *Eur. J. Pharm. Biopharm.* 81: 642–649.

Yamamoto, A., Takenouchi, K., and Ito, M. (1995). Impaired water barrier function in acne vulgaris. *Arch. Dermatol. Res.* 287: 214–218.

Yoshiike, T., Aikawa, Y., Sindhvananda, J., Suto, H., Nishimura, K., Kawamoto, T., and Ogawa, H. (1995). Skin barrier defect in atopic dermatitis: increased permeability of the stratum corneum using dimethyl sulfoxide and theophylline. *J. Dermatol. Sci.* 5: 92–96.

2 Theoretical Aspects of Transdermal and Topical Drug Delivery

2.1 TERMINOLOGY

Within the literature, there is variable use of terminology, acronyms, and abbreviations relating to transdermal and topical drug delivery. For clarity, the below defines terms used in this book:

Permeant: The molecular species that is moving into or through the skin.

Permeation: Movement of the drug *through* the membrane. This encompasses partitioning of the molecule into the various skin domains, such as into the stratum corneum intercellular lipids, and permeant diffusion through these domains.

Penetration: Entry of molecules into the skin. Penetration does not necessarily require the molecules to pass out of the tissue.

Diffusion: Movement of molecules through a domain, from high concentration (or high chemical potential) to low concentration (or low chemical potential), by random molecular movement.

Diffusivity: A property of the permeant in the membrane and a measure of how rapidly a permeant diffuses through the skin tissue. Diffusivity has S.I. units of m^2/s, but in permeation studies cm^2/h or cm^2/s are usually used.

Diffusion coefficient (D): The diffusion coefficient of the permeant, and a term used interchangeably with diffusivity. As with diffusivity, its common units are usually cm^2/h or cm^2/s.

Permeability coefficient (k_p): Essentially a measure of the speed of a permeant in the skin membrane, given in units of distance/time (usually cm/h). The permeability coefficient of a molecule is determined by its composition: for example, the molecule's molecular weight, the partition coefficient, the number of hydrogen bond donor and acceptors in the permeant.

Partition coefficient (P): A measure of the distribution of molecules between two phases. In transdermal (and many other) drug delivery studies, the partition coefficient between octanol and water is usually used as a guide for how well molecules will enter and traverse biological membranes. Due to the large numbers often encountered with partition coefficients, it is usual to quote log partition data. Two abbreviations are often used, K and P; in transdermal studies where k_p is used for the permeability coefficient, P is often the preferred abbreviation to minimise confusion.

Partitioning: The process of molecules distributing between two domains. In transdermal drug delivery work, partitioning is generally used to describe molecular redistribution from one domain to another, such as from an aqueous domain to a lipid domain.

Flux (J): The amount of permeant crossing the skin (or entering the systemic circulation). It is given in units of mass/area/time (usually $\mu g/cm^2/h$).

Membrane thickness (h): In various numerical treatments of permeation data, a term for the membrane thickness is required. This is problematic, since it is difficult to measure the skin membrane thickness during an experiment, and thickness will vary with the level of tissue hydration. Also, the barrier to permeation may reside solely in the stratum corneum or in the viable epidermal tissue or in a combination of both. Further, the pathway taken by a molecule across the tissue is seldom directly across the membrane, but a more tortuous route usually prevails for molecular movement through the stratum corneum. Again, a simple measure of membrane thickness is thus inappropriate. Several workers have estimated more reasonable pathlengths through the stratum corneum than a simple measure of thickness, as discussed in Section 2.3.3. In some older texts, the symbol δ is used to denote membrane thickness, but most modern texts have adopted the symbol h.

Lag time (L): Related to the period during which the rate of permeation across the membrane is increasing. It is obtained by extrapolating the pseudo steady-state portion of a plot of the cumulative amount traversing the membrane with time (see Figure 2.2). Clearly, if molecules bind to skin components during permeation, then their transport slows, and hence the lag time increases. Older texts have used the symbol τ whereas others have used t_L for the lag time, but most modern texts use the abbreviation L.

2.2   THE TRANSDERMAL PERMEATION PROCESS

There are multiple potential steps between a molecule's first application to the skin surface until it appears in the systemic circulation, and hence the permeation process is complex, as illustrated in Figure 2.1. Typically, the drug is applied to the skin in a vehicle (described in detail in Chapter 5). The vehicle may be simple, such as an aqueous solution, or it may be more complex, such as with an emulsion. The molecules adjacent to the stratum corneum surface will partition into the membrane dependent on their physicochemical properties. Thus, for a lipophilic molecule such as oestradiol (log $P_{(octanol/water)}$ = 2.29), partitioning into stratum corneum lipids from a saturated aqueous solution will be favourable. Clearly, when applied from an oily vehicle, the tendency for this steroid hormone to leave the vehicle will be lessened. In either case, the first step in transdermal delivery is partitioning of the therapeutic agent into the outermost layer of the stratum corneum. Since only molecules adjacent to the skin can partition from the vehicle into the tissue, further drug delivery is dependent upon molecules within the vehicle randomly redistributing to provide further molecules adjacent to the stratum corneum surface. Molecular diffusion through the vehicle again depends on the nature of the formulation (for example, its viscosity), and in some cases the diffusion of drug through the vehicle can limit

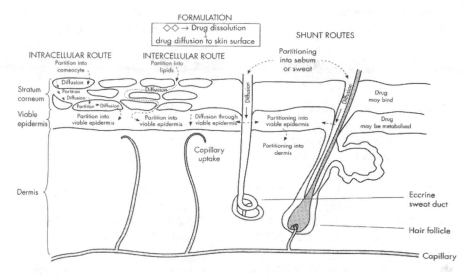

FIGURE 2.1 A representation of the principle mechanisms and pathways operating during transdermal and topical drug delivery. (From Williams, A.C., 2003. *Transdermal and Topical Drug Delivery*. London, UK: Pharmaceutical Press. With permission.)

the rate of transdermal drug delivery. Additional considerations will apply if the vehicle contains suspended particles. For poorly water-soluble drugs delivered from an aqueous system, dissolution of drug particles to maintain a saturated solution may be the rate-limiting step to transdermal drug delivery.

Once the permeant has partitioned into the outer layer of the stratum corneum, the drug then diffuses through the stratum corneum. This in itself may be a multi-step process, as parallel pathways for permeation exist (Section 2.3). At the stratum corneum/viable epidermis junction, there is another partitioning step as the molecules move into the viable tissue before further diffusion through the membrane to the epidermis/dermis junction. Again, there is partitioning followed by diffusion through the dermal tissue to the capillaries where there is another partitioning step for the molecules to enter the blood vessels before removal in the systemic circulation.

In addition to these multiple partitioning and diffusion processes for transdermal drug delivery, there are other potential fates for molecules entering human skin. Permeants may bind with various elements of the skin. For example, a drug binding to keratin within the stratum corneum could provide a reservoir effect. Further, excipients in topical formulations – such as solvents – will concomitantly penetrate into and permeate through the tissue which can alter the nature (solvating capacity) of, for example, the stratum corneum or its constituent domains. In addition, as described earlier, the skin is metabolically active and supports a wide range of bacterial and fungal species on its surface. The potential thus exists for drugs to be biotransformed prior to or during permeation; occasionally such biotransformations can be beneficial in allowing penetration of a lipophilic prodrug into the tissue with subsequent cleavage – often of an ester link – to liberate the active pharmaceutical agent. Further, depending on the nature of the drug, the permeant may not enter the systemic circulation but may partition into the subcutaneous fatty layer, and some molecules, for example, in liniment formulations, may even reach muscles.

2.3 PERMEATION PATHWAYS THROUGH THE STRATUM CORNEUM

It is generally acknowledged that the stratum corneum provides the principal rate-limiting barrier to topical and transdermal drug delivery. However, for some highly lipophilic drugs, partitioning out of the stratum corneum lipid domains into the essentially aqueous environment of the viable epidermis or dermis can become rate-limiting.

There are essentially three principal pathways by which a molecule can traverse intact stratum corneum: via the appendages (shunt routes), through the intercellular lipid domains, or by a transcellular route (Figure 2.1). It should be noted that the three different micro-routes are not mutually exclusive, and for any permeant ALL three (intercellular, intracellular, and shunt routes) operate, but the proportion of molecules crossing by the different routes will vary depending on the physicochemical properties of the permeant, as described in Section 2.4. Further, the presence of excipients and their own transport into – and interactions with – the stratum corneum can affect the nature of the three pathways.

2.3.1 TRANSAPPENDAGEAL TRANSPORT (SHUNT ROUTE TRANSPORT)

As described in Chapter 1, the dermis supports three skin appendages that extend to cross the stratum corneum barrier; the pilosebaceous unit, and the eccrine and apocrine ducts (see Sections 1.2.2.1, 1.2.2.2, and 1.2.2.3 respectively). These appendages offer a shunt route (or "short-cut") by which molecules could enter the lower layers of the skin without having to traverse the barrier provided by the stratum corneum.

In practice, the surface openings provide only a small fraction of the total skin surface area. For example, on the forearm, hair follicles occupy approximately 0.1% of the surface area, although on the forehead, this may be as much as 13% (Otberg et al., 2004). The density of eccrine sweat glands also varies significantly with body site. Approximately 250 eccrine glands are found per cm^2 of the volar aspect of the hand (the palm) and ~300 per cm^2 on the volar aspect of the foot (sole), in contrast to ~100 per cm^2 on the cheek or lateral thigh (Taylor and Machado-Moreira, 2013). However, the eccrine duct openings onto the skin surface are relatively small and the ducts are either evacuated or are actively secreting sweat that would be expected to diminish inward diffusion of topically applied agents. The opening of the follicular pore to the skin surface is considerably larger than that of the eccrine glands, though they are less numerous. The duct of the sebaceous gland is again filled, but rather than aqueous sweat, the sebum in these follicular glands is lipoidal.

It is rather simplistic to view the shunt routes as insignificant for most permeants; the shunt routes were shown to be minor, yet significant, contributors (5–10%) in the steady-state flux of steroids through excised human skin (Siddiqui et al., 1989). In order to determine the relative contribution of the shunt routes to drug delivery, a "skin sandwich" model was developed (El Maghraby et al., 2001; Essa et al., 2002).

In essence, a human epidermal membrane, prepared from abdominal tissue, is overlaid with a second membrane of human stratum corneum. This doubles the thickness of the skin barrier (the stratum corneum) but, given the relatively low surface area of the shunts on the abdomen, it is unlikely that the shunt route openings would align, and the top layer of stratum corneum blocks most of the shunts available in the lower membrane (Figure 2.2).

If the shunt routes are not involved in permeation, then since the steady-state flux of a drug through the skin is inversely proportional to the membrane thickness ($J \propto h^{-1}$, described in detail below), doubling the effective thickness of the principal barrier – the stratum corneum – is expected to halve the steady-state flux of the permeant through the sandwich. Likewise, since the lag time to pseudo steady-state flux is directly proportional to the thickness squared ($L \propto h^2$), then the lag time is expected to be prolonged 4-fold. Using this protocol, the steady-state flux of oestradiol from a saturated aqueous solution reduced by 57% through the sandwich model compared to flux through a single epidermal membrane, in good agreement with the anticipated 50% reduction, illustrating that this lipophilic drug permeates predominantly through the bulk stratum corneum (El Maghraby et al., 2001). In contrast, using the same model, Essa et al. (2002) showed that for mannitol, flux was essentially blocked for the first nine hours of application to the skin sandwich, whereas drug delivery through a single membrane was seen. These data clearly show a major role for the shunt routes in transdermal delivery of this hydrophilic molecule. Also noteworthy was that, as the experiment was prolonged, mannitol was subsequently detected in

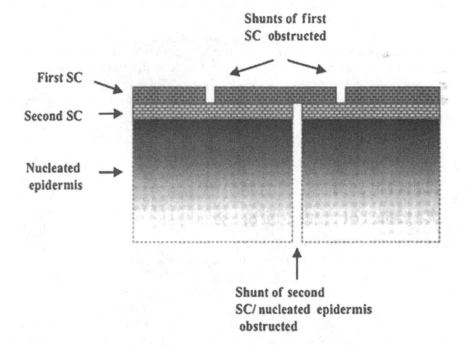

FIGURE 2.2 The skin sandwich model showing the obstruction of the shunt routes in the lower epidermal skin sample by an overlaid additional stratum corneum membrane.

the receiving solution, indicating that whilst the shunt routes may dominate, some transport through the bulk stratum corneum occurred. An alternative approach to assess transappendageal transport was taken by Teichmann et al. (2005a) who used a varnish–wax mixture to selectively block follicles. Subsequently, a "differential stripping" approach was used to remove permeants from the bulk stratum corneum by sequentially removing layers of the stratum corneum by tape stripping, followed by extraction of material within follicles using cyanoacrylate glue (Teichmann et al., 2005b; Ossadnik et al., 2007).

When using "standard" skin membranes, the relative contribution of the shunt routes to drug flux can be affected by experimental design – *in vivo*/*in vitro* tissue, animal or human skin, finite or infinite dosing, pseudo steady-state or transient measurements. For example, water content of the stratum corneum is known to affect diffusivity; as the tissue hydrates, its permeability to most drugs increases. To avoid alterations in the stratum corneum water content during experiments, as may happen if applying an aqueous drug solution, most researchers ensure full tissue hydration prior to the experiment. However, hydrating the membrane can have other consequences. For example, the skin swells, and as it does so, it is likely that the shunt route openings onto the skin surface are constricted. Thus, *in vitro* experiments with fully hydrated stratum corneum may obscure the influence of transappendageal transport. Similarly, many *in vitro* experiments examine pseudo steady-state flux, where the shunt route contribution may well be low. However, with finite dosing and at short time periods after drug application, the relative contribution of the shunt route pathway may be considerably greater, since molecules will not have had time to traverse the bulk of the stratum corneum.

In addition to initial rapid drug delivery, and the greater significance *in vivo* than *in vitro*, transappendageal transport may also be important for large polar molecules and ions that would traverse poorly across the bulk of the stratum corneum. The shunt routes are also important for delivering vesicular structures to the skin and for targeting their contents to the pilosebaceous units; there is considerable debate as to whether vesicles can traverse the stratum corneum intact, but a strong body of evidence shows that these structures can penetrate into the pilosebaceous units (Lauer et al., 1996).

Much effort has been devoted to developing micro- and nano-sized carriers to target delivery to follicles, and to form depots for prolonged release of drugs, such as adapalene to treat acne. In addition to liposomes, follicular targeting using solid-lipid nanoparticles, polymeric particles, and dendrimer materials have been explored. Delivery into follicles has been reported for carriers ranging from 20 nm diameters up to 800 nm (e.g., Toll et al., 2004), and to significant depths within the tissue. It is clear that delivery of these carriers into the follicles is mechanically supported, an effect that may not be seen in excised tissue. Micro- and nanoparticles applied to the skin surface tend to accumulate at the follicular openings. The cuticle of the hair shaft has a zig-zag structure along its length. *In vivo*, the hairs are continually moving and act as a "geared pump" moving the particles deeper into the follicular duct (Lademann et al., 2007). Such endogenous movement is difficult to replicate *in vitro*, even with rubbing of systems onto the excised skin surface, and may explain discrepancies between *in vivo* and *in vitro* results of particulate delivery to follicles.

Vesicles (Section 4.2) and nano-carriers (Section 4.3) are described in further detail in Chapter 4.

Iontophoretic drug delivery uses electrical charge to drive molecules into the skin. This process also largely depends on the presence of shunt routes; charge is carried through the stratum corneum via the path of least resistance, and the shunt routes provide less resistance than the stratum corneum bulk. These (and other) drug delivery technologies are described in Chapter 4.

2.3.2 Transcellular Route

The transcellular ("through the cells"; also known as intracellular) pathway for a permeant to cross the intact stratum corneum is often regarded as a polar or hydrophilic route through the membrane. As described in Chapter 1 (Section 1.2.3.6), the stratum corneum corneocytes are predominantly filled with tight bundles of intracellular keratin which is hydrated, and so apparently provides an essentially aqueous environment for diffusion of hydrophilic molecules. However, corneocytes are bounded by a cornified cell envelope of covalently cross-linked proteins and covalently bound lipids, and then connected to the intercellular multiply bilayered lipid domains.

Consequently, any permeant crossing intact stratum corneum via the transcellular route faces numerous repeating hurdles. Firstly, the molecule will enter the hydrated corneocyte according to its partition coefficient; this will be favoured by hydrophilic molecules with a log $P_{octanol/water}$ typically <1. After entry, the molecule will diffuse through the corneocyte, driven by a concentration gradient across the cell. In order to leave the cell, the molecule must enter the bilayer lipids, which will be favourable for lipophilic molecules with a log $P_{octanol/water}$ typically >1, before diffusion through the lipid lamella to reach the next corneocyte. Conceptually, there are even greater levels of complexity in the environments that a molecule encounters. As shown in Figure 1.4 (Chapter 1), the lipid domains are themselves complex with hydrophobic chains and hydrophilic head groups (with associated water). Again, there will be multiple partitioning and diffusion steps within the 4 to 20 bilayer lipid lamellae between the corneocytes. Clearly, the multiple alternating hydrophilic and lipophilic domains that would be encountered via the transcellular route provide a significant obstacle for a permeant with defined physicochemical properties such as its fixed partition coefficient.

Despite the above, transcellular permeation cannot be ignored, in particular for highly hydrophilic permeants. Sznitowska et al. (1998) showed that polar lipids within the intercellular bilayers provided the principal barrier to baclofen (a hydrophilic zwitterion) permeating through skin since extraction of these lipids increased flux dramatically, whereas removal of less polar lipids caused minimal drug flux increases. The authors also note that intra- and intercellular permeation (and transport via the shunt routes) operate concomitantly. More recently, Miller et al. (2017) evaluated uptake and desorption of varied hydrophilic materials in human stratum corneum. The experimental data was fitted to a transcellular diffusion model which involved hindered diffusion of highly hydrophilic species through lipid defects and/ or desmosomes that connect the corneocytes. However, the authors also noted that it is highly likely that skin appendages play a role in both transient and steady-state absorption of hydrophilic compounds. Further, detailed modelling into the effects of stratum corneum heterogeneity, anisotropy, asymmetry, and follicular pathway on transdermal permeation of diethyl phthalate, caffeine, and nicotine concluded that diffusion is primarily transcellular and that the main barrier is located in the lipid layers (Barbero and Frasch, 2017).

The nature of the permeant will influence the relative importance of the transcellular route to the observed flux; for highly hydrophilic molecules, the transcellular route may predominate at pseudo steady state. However, the rate-limiting barrier for permeation via this route remains the multiply bilayered lipids that the molecule must traverse between the keratinocytes; the use of solvents to remove lipids from the stratum corneum invariably increases drug flux for even highly hydrophilic molecules. It should also be borne in mind that in addition to permeation via the transcellular route, the keratin also provides potential binding sites for solutes.

2.3.3 INTERCELLULAR PATHWAY

The lipid bilayers comprise around 1% of the stratum corneum diffusional area yet provide the only continuous phase within the membrane. There continues to be debate regarding the relative contributions of the intercellular and transcellular pathways for drug permeation; in essence, the relative proportion of a permeant traversing via these (and the shunt) routes is dependent on the molecule's physicochemical properties, its formulation, and dosing. For lipophilic permeants, it may be anticipated that the lipid domains provide a more suitable environment into which they enter the tissue than the essentially aqueous domains of the corneocytes.

The importance of the stratum corneum lipids in regulating the loss of water from the body and in controlling the penetration of materials into the skin has long been established. Following perturbation of the intercellular lipids by, for example, penetration enhancers, or their removal by solvents, transepidermal water loss increases and the flux of most permeants increases through delipidised skin. However, removal or perturbation of the intercellular lipids would generally increase flux via both intercellular and transcellular pathways.

Again, it is a gross simplification to merely describe the stratum corneum lipids as multiple bilayers. As described in Chapter 1 (Figure 1.4), the composition of these bilayers is uniquely different to all other lipid membrane bilayers within the body; notably, phospholipids are absent and varied ceramides are present. As well as the unique composition, stratum corneum lipids exist in a variety of states: a highly ordered and densely packed orthorhombic phase which is crystalline and exhibits low permeability to drug molecules, an ordered less densely packed, gel-like, more permeable hexagonal phase, and a disordered, highly permeable liquid phase. Further, there are likely regions of lipid "defects", perhaps accentuated where desmosomes connect corneocytes. The lipid bilayers thus offer multiple domains into which drugs of differing physicochemical properties can distribute and through which they can diffuse.

The precise nature of the intercellular pathway is still open to debate. What is clear, however, is that the multiple lipid bilayers provide the major limiting barrier to the flux of most drugs; intercellular transport is predominantly via the lipid domains, but intracellular permeation also requires the lipid lamellae to be crossed. With intracellular permeation, the pathway is regarded as being directly across the stratum corneum, and hence the pathlength for permeation is usually taken as the thickness of the stratum corneum. In contrast, the intercellular route is highly tortuous, with permeants moving through the continuous lipid domains between the corneocytes. In this case, the pathlength taken by the molecule is considerably greater than that of the stratum corneum thickness. Various estimates have been proposed for the intercellular permeation distance, ranging from 150 to 500 μm; it appears likely that different pathlengths are taken by permeants traversing the stratum corneum, dependent upon their physicochemical properties. As the real pathlength is unknown, various permeation parameters incorporating length (such as the permeability coefficient and diffusion coefficient) should always be regarded as *apparent* values.

2.4 INFLUENCE OF PERMEANT PHYSICOCHEMICAL PROPERTIES ON ROUTE OF ABSORPTION

From the above, it is clear that the relative contribution of the three potential pathways through the stratum corneum will vary depending on the nature of the permeant. The following properties will influence the permeation process, but it is again worth emphasising that all permeants are expected to utilise – to some extent – all three of the pathways outlined above.

2.4.1 PARTITION COEFFICIENT

When applied to the outer surface of the skin, a permeant will enter the stratum corneum according to its partition coefficient. Indeed, uptake into the tissue (often termed "partitioning" into the skin) could be the rate-limiting step in the permeation process. The partition coefficient of a permeant usually dictates the pathway that it primarily follows through the skin. Rather simplistically, it may be expected that a hydrophilic molecule will partition preferentially into the hydrated keratin-filled keratinocytes rather than into the lipid bilayers, whereas lipophilic permeants will preferentially partition into the lipoidal domains. Consequently, hydrophilic molecules may permeate largely via the intracellular route, whereas the intercellular route will often dominate for lipophilic molecules.

With a homologous series of permeants, there have been numerous studies over many years showing that increasing lipophilicity – for example, by increasing the alkyl chain length – increases flux (e.g., Flynn and Yalkowski, 1972). Thus, it follows that the bilayered lipids are rate-limiting in lipophilic permeant flux, and that the partition coefficient has allowed permeation predominantly via the intercellular route. However, the situation is not as clear for hydrophilic permeants. As previously described, the intercellular route is not exclusively lipoidal – there are desmosomes and proteins associated with the lipid domains, and a thin layer of water is found between the polar head groups in the lipid bilayers – and it is feasible that a hydrophilic permeant may partition into these more polar areas within the lipid bilayers, and hence also traverse the tissue via the intercellular route. Given these biological complexities, the "mixed permeation model" describes that most drugs permeate largely via the continuous intercellular lipid domains, but both the lipid and polar regions of the bilayers could provide the micro-routes, depending on the partition coefficient of the permeant (Roberts et al., 1995).

For molecules with intermediate partition coefficients, showing some solubility in both oil and water phases, the intercellular route probably predominates. This would typically encompass most molecules with a log $P_{(octanol/water)}$ of approximately 1–4. For more highly lipophilic molecules (log P >4), the intercellular route will be almost exclusively the pathway used to traverse the stratum corneum. However, for these molecules, a further consideration is the ability to partition out of the stratum corneum into the essentially aqueous viable epidermal tissues, a factor that is expanded upon with respect to experimental design in Chapter 6. For more hydrophilic molecules (log P <1), the transcellular route becomes increasingly important, yet there are still lipid bilayers to cross between the keratinocytes. For highly hydrophilic (and charged) molecules, the appendageal pathway may also become significant, as is shown by the localisation around the pilosebaceous units of topically applied dyes.

2.4.2 MOLECULAR SIZE

A second major factor in determining the flux of a material through human skin is the size and shape of the molecule. When considering the influence of molecular size on permeation, molecular volume is the most appropriate measure of permeant bulk. However, for simplicity, the molecular weight is generally taken as an approximation of molecular volume, with an inherent assumption that most molecules are essentially spherical.

It has long been appreciated that, in simple isotropic media, molecular weight influences the diffusion coefficient of a molecule, with increasingly bulky molecules showing decreasing diffusivities (Crank, 1975). Despite the heterogeneity within human skin, this relationship also exists. However, most conventional therapeutic agents (small organic molecules) that are selected as candidates for transdermal delivery tend to lie within a relatively narrow range of molecular weights (100–500 Da). Within such a narrow range, the influence of molecular weight on drug flux appears to be relatively minor if compared to the influence of, for example, changes in partition coefficients.

It is evident that most commercially successful topical and transdermal products contain active ingredients with a molecular weight of <500 Da: for example, oestradiol (272 Da), fentanyl (336 Da), and nicotine (162 Da). Though there are a few exceptions, such as the macrolactam immunosuppressives pimecrolimus (810 Da) and tacrolimus (804 Da) that are used topically to treat atopic dermatitis, the commercial and experimental data "has led to the so-called '500 Dalton Rule', which states that for a drug to be deliverable through native skin, it must have a molecular weight of less than 500 Daltons ..." (Bos and Meinardi, 2000). However, there is a growing body of evidence showing that larger molecular weight biomacromolecules are able to penetrate into, and to some extent, diffuse through, human skin (see Section 2.4.6).

2.4.3 SOLUBILITY/MELTING POINT

It is well known that most organic materials with high melting points and high enthalpies of melting have relatively low aqueous solubilities at normal temperatures and pressures (i.e., under the typical conditions in transdermal drug delivery). Thus, there is a clear relationship between melting point and solubility and there are several theoretical models available that predict solubilities from melting point data.

From the discussion of the intercellular permeation pathway above (Section 2.3.3), it is clear that lipophilic molecules tend to permeate through the skin faster – have shorter lag times – than more hydrophilic molecules. Thus, solubility within the intercellular lipids (usually described by the partition coefficient) can be correlated with the permeability coefficient for a homologous series of compounds. However, whilst moderately high lipophilicity is generally a desirable (or required) feature of transdermal candidates, it is also necessary for the molecule to exhibit some aqueous solubility since topical medicaments are often applied from an aqueous formulation and the deeper layers of the skin are more hydrophilic. Indeed, the steady-state flux of a drug traversing the tissue is the product of the permeability coefficient and the applied concentration (Section 2.5.1). Whilst lipophilic permeants may provide a relatively high permeability coefficient, their lipophilicity will usually dictate that the aqueous solubility (and hence concentration in an aqueous formulation) will be relatively low, with a consequent impact upon drug flux through the tissue.

One further factor to consider is the potential for depletion of the permeant from a donor system. If the drug has poor water solubility, and is delivered from a saturated or sub-saturated aqueous formulation, then the amount of drug present in the formulation will be relatively low. As a lipophilic permeant, the molecule will rapidly enter the stratum corneum, which could quickly deplete the drug within the formulation. As the concentration of the drug falls, so the thermodynamic activity of the drug in the formulation will fall and hence the driving force for diffusion drops and consequently the flux will rapidly decrease.

As with most of the formulation factors within the field of transdermal drug delivery, a compromise in candidate solubility properties is thus required. Some drug lipophilicity is desirable, allowing uptake into the stratum corneum and transport through the intercellular lipids, yet with some aqueous solubility to provide enough permeant within an aqueous formulation to minimise the effect of donor depletion over the time course of application.

2.4.4 IONISATION

Considering the nature of the stratum corneum barrier to transdermal delivery, residing largely within the lipid bilayer domains, it is widely believed that ionisable drugs are poor transdermal permeants. Indeed, many of the arguments against using weak acids and weak bases that will dissociate to varying degrees depending on the pH of the formulation (and on the pH of the stratum corneum) are founded in the pH-partition hypothesis. According to this hypothesis, developed for absorption of drugs through the gastrointestinal tract, only the un-ionised form of the drug can permeate the lipid barrier in significant amounts. However, with the complex structure of human skin, this model cannot be rigidly applied, and it is notable that many drugs under development for topical and transdermal use are weak acids or weak bases.

As described above, permeation across human skin can be via several pathways, none of which are mutually exclusive, and all of which probably operate for most molecules traversing the skin. Some appendages offer an essentially aqueous pathway through the stratum corneum, albeit one of limited cross-sectional area. The transcellular route can be considered to possess intermediate properties, whereas the intercellular pathway is essentially a lipophilic route. Thus, it is likely that charged permeants (ionised drugs) can cross the membrane by the shunt route, but that their permeability coefficient may be significantly lower than if the species were un-ionised and were to pass largely via the lipoidal intercellular route. Indeed, electrically assisted transdermal drug delivery essentially drives ions – iontophoresis – through the shunt routes (Section 4.7.1).

Further complexity can be introduced if one considers the relative aqueous solubilities of the ionised and un-ionised species. As described in Section 2.5.1 (Equation 2.9), drug flux is the product of the permeability coefficient and effective drug concentration in the vehicle. Although the permeability coefficient of the un-ionised species through the lipid membrane may be high, its aqueous solubility could be low. In contrast, for an ionised species, then the permeability coefficient may be low, but the aqueous solubility will likely be high. It is conceivable that the resultant fluxes from these two situations may be equivalent, and hence the simplistic "rule" that only un-ionised species can be effectively delivered into and through skin must be regarded with significant caution.

2.4.5   Other Factors

The literature contains various predictive models for estimating transdermal drug flux. The majority of these models use simple inputs: drug aqueous solubility, melting point, molecular weight, and partition coefficient (usually octanol/water). However, beyond these four prime determinants of permeant flux, there are other molecular properties that can affect drug delivery through the skin.

Drug-binding is a factor that should be borne in mind when selecting appropriate candidates. Considering the varied nature of skin components (lipids, proteins, aqueous regions, enzymes, etc.) and the variety within permeants (weak acids/bases, ionised species, neutral molecules, etc.), there are numerous potential interactions between drug substances and the tissue. Interactions can vary from hydrogen bonding to weak Van der Waals forces, and the result of drug-binding (if any) on flux across the tissue will vary depending on the permeant. For example, with a poorly water-soluble drug in an aqueous donor solution (thus containing relatively few drug molecules), significant binding to the stratum corneum may completely retard drug flux if essentially all the molecules entering the tissue from the donor solution bind to skin components. In contrast, for molecules with moderate water solubility that permeate the skin well, binding sites within the tissue may be occupied during the early periods of transdermal delivery and hence, with occupied binding sites, steady-state flux may be unaffected.

One important consequence of binding between the applied drug and skin components is the effect on lag time. There is a delay between applying a drug to the outer surface of the tissue and its appearance in a receptor solution (if performing an *in vitro* experiment) or the blood (*in vivo*). This delay, resulting from the time taken for the molecules to traverse the stratum corneum/skin membrane is related to the lag time; pseudo steady-state flux prevails after approximately 2.7 times the lag time. If the drug binds during its passage through the tissue, then the lag time will clearly be prolonged. For steady-state drug delivery, as with, for example, hormone replacement patch therapy, then this increase in time taken to achieve therapeutic levels is seldom important. However, if a drug such as hydrocortisone is applied from a finite dose, where the formulation may be rubbed into a site for typically <1 minute before excess medicament is removed, then the delay and reduced availability from the applied dose due to drug/skin binding may be more significant.

The influence of hydrogen bond activity of applied therapeutic agents on drug flux has been investigated in some detail, but there remains debate as to the hydrogen bonding nature of the stratum corneum and whether it is a predominantly hydrogen bond donating or accepting medium. However, it is clear that diffusion through human epidermal membranes is not dependent solely upon the number of hydrogen bonding groups in a molecule per se, but also upon their distribution with respect to symmetry within the molecule. From the above, it is apparent that permeation across the stratum corneum can be dramatically reduced by increasing the number of hydrogen bonding groups on the permeant.

Binding of a drug to stratum corneum components can form a reservoir of the drug from which delivery can be prolonged over extended periods of time. Indeed, over 50 years ago, Vickers (1963) demonstrated that a topically applied corticosteroid formed a reservoir that remained in the stratum corneum for many days. Whilst a reservoir can form through drug–skin binding, the delivery of excipients, and in particular solvents, into the stratum corneum from topical formulations can also form a drug reservoir within the tissue.

Depending on the type of formulation selected, other factors may be important in a transdermal delivery system. For example, if the drug is suspended, then the particle size may become a key regulator of flux; if the drug has a low solubility in the vehicle and dissolution of the particles is thus rate-limiting in flux, then decreasing the particle size will increase drug dissolution rate in the vehicle and hence promote transdermal delivery. If a drug is racemic, it may be possible to improve delivery by selection of lowest melting (i.e., highest solubility) enantiomers, as was shown for the chiral β-blockers atenolol, alprenolol, and propranolol delivered across cadaver skin (Touitou et al., 1994). Racemic propranolol has a 21°C higher melting point than its enantiomer which resulted in a 3-fold higher flux for the S – (-) form compared to the racemate. Considering that the pure enantiomer has a 2-order of magnitude greater pharmacological activity than the racemate, this relatively modest flux increase could be clinically significant. Similarly, delivery of chiral terpene penetration enhancers has been improved through selection of the lower melting form (Mackay et al., 2001). The effects of melting point depression on drug delivery to and through the skin are considered further in Section 3.4.3.

2.4.6 BIOMACROMOLECULES

It should be noted that the physicochemical determinants of flux described above relate to "conventional" small molecule active pharmaceutical ingredients and reflect the properties of current commercially successful formulations. However, there is a growing body of evidence, supported by advances in assay sensitivity, to show that some larger biomacromolecules may passively penetrate into intact, as well as diseased, human skin. These include peptides and proteins, recombinant antibodies, antisense oligonucleotides, and aptamers. For these, whilst rates of penetration into and permeation through skin may be extremely low, their high potencies may elicit pharmacological activity.

Hyaluronic acid is a hygroscopic macromolecule widely used in topical formulations (Brown and Jones, 2005). Recently, its uptake into human stratum corneum has been studied using Raman spectroscopy, illustrating that, in violation of the 500 Da "rule", the polymer with molecular weights of 20–50,000 Da penetrated into the stratum corneum, and was visualised in deeper skin layers (Essendoubi et al., 2016).

Short-interfering RNAs (siRNAs) offer potential tools to treat common skin disorders, but as negatively charged, hydrophilic, and typically large (~13–14 kDa) molecules, their topical delivery is challenging. However, using a range of penetration enhancement strategies, including conjugation to SPACE-Peptide (Hsu and Mitragotri, 2011) coupled with an ethosome-based carrier, showed delivery of the peptide into mouse skin (Chen et al., 2014). Whilst naked siRNA (and miRNA) do not appear to effectively enter the stratum corneum, chemical modification not only improves RNA stability but can also facilitate uptake into the tissue (Hedge et al., 2014).

Recently, we demonstrated passive aptamer delivery into intact human skin (Lenn et al., 2018). Aptamers are a relatively new class of oligonucleotide-based molecules that can specifically bind to target molecules, including proteins or other cellular targets; aptamers have been approved for macular degeneration, and new aptamers are in clinical development for cancer, haemophilia, anaemia, and diabetes. We developed and optimised a first-in-class RNA aptamer inhibitor of IL-23 for topical treatment of psoriasis. The 62-nucleotide (20,395 Da) aptamer had high affinity and specificity to human IL-23 cytokine. Employing a well-validated *in vitro* human skin model to assess topical delivery, we showed for the first time that *without* physically disrupting the stratum corneum, this large molecular weight biomacromolecule penetrated into and permeated through human skin, and elicited a biological response. Again confounding the "500 Da rule" and the molecular weight considerations described above for conventional "small" permeants, RNA aptamer variants whose molecular weights ranged from 12.5 to 29.3 kDA (36- to 85-mers) all penetrated into intact human skin and their fluorescence signals were visualised within the epidermis. There was no evidence to show that delivery was primarily via the shunt routes, and a single domain antibody fragment (13.1 kDa) was not able to penetrate into the epidermis.

With increasingly sophisticated and sensitive assays being developed for varied biomacromolecule drugs, and given their high potencies and specificities (requiring low dosages at their target sites), it appears likely that greater numbers of these therapeutic agents will be developed for topical delivery. However, the mechanisms by which these agents traverse the stratum corneum barrier remain unclear. It may be anticipated that the primary pathway is via shunt route delivery and subsequent lateral diffusion through the more hydrophilic epidermal and dermal domains. However, in our aptamer study, we saw no evidence for localisation of the permeant around the follicles.

2.5 MATHEMATICS OF SKIN PERMEATION

Human skin is a multiply layered, complex, heterogeneous biological tissue that varies enormously from person to person and site to site. It thus appears unrealistic to attempt to describe the behaviour of such a system with ideal mathematical models. However, despite these complexities, relatively simple mathematical treatments, such as Fick's second law of diffusion, can be applied to data obtained from experiments with human skin. Drug absorption across human skin is passive (to date, no active transport mechanisms have been reported) and hence can be described in physical terms. The following description of the mathematical treatments applied to transdermal drug delivery studies is intended to provide an overview. Only two situations will be considered:

1. Where the drug is applied as an infinite dose – it does not deplete over the time of application (e.g., as with a transdermal patch)
2. Where a small finite dose is applied and so pseudo steady-state permeation would not be encountered (e.g., with a cream for a local action)

For more detailed treatments of diffusional phenomena, the reader is urged to consult the excellent book by Crank (1975) in which equations are derived for various experimental designs that are occasionally employed in transdermal drug delivery studies.

2.5.1 PSEUDO STEADY-STATE PERMEATION (INFINITE DOSING)

The amount of a material passing through a unit area per unit time is termed the flux (J). The molecules move in response to a thermodynamic force arising from a concentration gradient. Fick's first law of diffusion states that the rate of transfer of the diffusing substance through the unit area of a section is proportional to the concentration gradient measured normal to the section. We can write:

$$J = -D\frac{\delta C}{\delta x} \tag{2.1}$$

where J is the flux of the permeant per unit area, D is the diffusion coefficient of the permeant, and $\delta C/\delta x$ is the concentration gradient (C is the concentration and x is the space coordinate measured normal to the section).

Fick's second law of diffusion can be derived from Equation 2.1. When a topically applied permeant enters the skin, it is usually assumed that diffusion is unidirectional (i.e., that the concentration gradient is from the outer surface into the tissue). Unidirectional diffusion in an isotropic medium is expressed mathematically by Fick's second law of diffusion:

$$\frac{\delta C}{\delta t} = D \frac{\delta^2 C}{\delta x^2} \tag{2.2}$$

where t is time. Thus, the rate of change in concentration with time at a point within a diffusional field is proportional to the rate of change in the concentration gradient at that point.

Mathematical treatments of permeation data use Fick's second law of diffusion and solve it with the conditions appropriate for the experimental protocol, considering geometry, boundary conditions, initial conditions, and so on. However, the skin membrane is highly complex, and hence precise mathematical solutions to permeation data are not possible. For example, different skin membranes are often used (stratum corneum alone, or entire epidermis comprising stratum corneum and viable epidermis, or dermal membranes) and multiple pathways for permeation may operate at one time (appendageal, intercellular, and transcellular). Thus, the following solutions to Fick's second law must be treated as useful approximations that allow comparisons and standardisation of permeation data.

Most *in vitro* experimental designs aim to mimic as closely as possible the *in vivo* situation. The most common *in vitro* design is one where a membrane (usually the epidermis or a dermatomed section with the epidermis and some dermal tissue) separates two compartments. One compartment contains the permeant in a vehicle, possibly a simple aqueous or buffer solution (termed the donor solution), and the other compartment contains a receptor (or receiver) solution that provides sink conditions (i.e., essentially zero concentration). After sufficient time, pseudo steady-state permeation across the membrane is achieved when the concentration gradient of the permeant across the membrane is constant. Under these conditions, Equation 2.2 can be simplified to:

$$\frac{dM}{dt} = \text{flux}(J) = \frac{DC_0}{h} \tag{2.3}$$

where M is the cumulative mass of permeant that passes through per unit area of the membrane in time t; dM/dt is the rate of change of cumulative mass of permeant that passes per unit area through the membrane, usually termed the flux (J) of the permeant. C_0 is the concentration of the permeant in the first layer of the membrane (at the skin surface, in contact with the donor solution), and h is the membrane thickness.

In practical terms, it is very difficult to measure C_0, the concentration of permeant in the first layer of the membrane; removal of the outer layer for assay is problematic, and contamination from the applied donor solution is almost inevitable. However, the concentration of the permeant in the vehicle (donor solution) bathing the skin membrane (C_v) is usually known or can be determined relatively easily. Since C_0 and C_v are simply related by:

$$P = C_0 / C_v \quad \text{so} \quad C_0 = PC_v \tag{2.4}$$

where P is the partition coefficient of the permeant between the membrane and the vehicle. Substitution of Equation 2.4 into Equation 2.3 gives:

$$\frac{dM}{dt} = J = \frac{DPC_v}{h} \tag{2.5}$$

This is a widely applied equation used to analyse transdermal drug delivery data. A plot of M, the cumulative amount of drug passing through a unit area of membrane (e.g., $\mu g/cm^2$) against time gives the typical permeation profile reported in most investigations, as shown in Figure 2.3.

The lag time can be obtained from extrapolation of the pseudo steady-state portion of the permeation profile to the intercept on the time axis. As a useful approximation, pseudo steady-state permeation for most drugs is achieved after around 2.7 times the lag time (Barry, 1983). Crank (1975) showed that the lag time (L) can be related to the diffusion coefficient by:

$$L = \frac{h^2}{6D} \tag{2.6}$$

Equation 2.6 shows that it is feasible to determine the diffusion coefficient of a molecule in the membrane by measuring the lag time. Indeed, this approach has been used for studies with simple isotropic physical membranes such as polymers. However, skin is not a simple isotropic membrane. As described above, difficulties are encountered when measuring the membrane thickness: is the rate determining barrier the stratum corneum alone, or does it include the viable epidermal tissue?

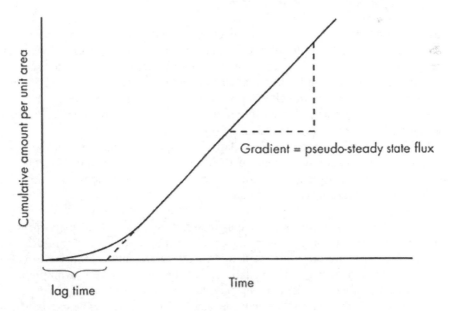

FIGURE 2.3 Typical permeation profile for an infinite dose application to human skin membranes.

Application of various vehicles can expand the membrane, and indeed, a simple measure of thickness does not account for the tortuous intercellular pathway for diffusion. As the membrane thickness is a squared factor in Equation 2.6, any minor errors in this parameter rapidly magnify. Additionally, lag times obtained from permeation experiments with human skin tend to be highly variable and can be strongly influenced by permeant–skin binding.

An alternative approach to determine the apparent diffusion coefficient of a permeant from a pseudo steady-state permeation profile requires rearrangement of Equation 2.5 to:

$$D = \frac{Jh}{PC_v} \quad\quad (2.7)$$

This expression allows calculation of the apparent diffusion coefficient without requiring an accurate lag time value, but does still require an approximation for the membrane thickness (though not squared). The partition coefficient (stratum corneum/vehicle) for the permeant can be obtained from separate experimentation.

Because of the difficulty in accurately assessing membrane thickness, a composite parameter, the permeability coefficient (k_p) is often used and is given as:

$$k_p = \frac{PD}{h} \quad\quad (2.8)$$

which can be substituted into Equation 2.5 to give:

$$J = k_p C_v \qu\quad (2.9)$$

The pseudo steady-state flux, J, is simply obtained as the gradient of the linear portion of the permeation profile (Figure 2.3), and if the concentration of the permeant in the applied vehicle is known, then the permeability coefficient can be determined. It is this parameter, the permeability coefficient, which is often used to characterise the permeation of drugs through skin; other parameters such as the diffusion coefficient can be used, but are more difficult to calculate accurately due to difficulties estimating, for example, membrane thickness.

Though the above equations are relatively simple and easy to use, there are some important assumptions made in their derivations. The validity of some of the assumptions is questionable, and for some experimental designs, the equations become invalid. Thus, it is assumed that:

1. The stratum corneum is the major rate-limiting barrier, and the primary rate-determining step is permeation through the stratum corneum and not partitioning into or out of the membrane. This assumption appears to be valid for most permeants, though for very lipophilic or very hydrophilic molecules, then partitioning behaviour may become rate-limiting.
2. Permeation through the appendages (shunt routes) is negligible compared to permeation through the bulk of the stratum corneum. This will be the case for most permeants, but for ions and large molecules, the shunt routes

may be highly significant. Clearly, the above equations only apply at pseudo steady state and do not hold for permeation during the early time course of the process.

3. Permeation through the stratum corneum is solely by passive diffusion. To date, no active transport mechanisms have been reported.

4. The nature of the stratum corneum is not altered by the application of the vehicle. This is clearly not the case if dry (or partially hydrated) stratum corneum is used as the membrane and an aqueous donor solution is applied. Similarly, some vehicles (such as propylene glycol) have been shown to partition into the stratum corneum, thus altering the solvent nature of the tissue and hence affecting partitioning of the permeant into the membrane.

5. The drug is in solution within the stratum corneum. Given the varied nature of the tissue, this appears a reasonable assumption for most drugs.

6. The diffusion coefficient of the permeant is independent of concentration, time, or distance. This is a questionable assumption, since many permeants would be expected to bind to some extent to the tissue, effectively making diffusion coefficients dependent upon concentration. Additionally, permeants may exist in different states of self-association dependent upon the applied concentration – dimethyl sulphoxide can exist in many self-assembled states, including dimers and hydrates, depending on the environment in which it is placed. Thus, the diffusion coefficients calculated from transdermal permeation experiments must be regarded as *apparent* diffusion coefficients, since the errors inherent in using the above equations prevent absolute values from being generated.

7. Equation 2.6 (relating lag time to diffusion coefficient) is only applicable to situations where there is no binding between the permeant and the tissue.

8. Fickian diffusion theory was developed for isotropic media. The stratum corneum is a heterogeneous membrane, yet we assume that it is uniform in character.

Despite these caveats, it is surprising that such simple equations fit experimental skin permeation data so well. More complex models and equations have been developed, some mathematically based, others using simulated data or compartmentalised models. However, the majority of literature reports use Fickian theory to describe experimental data and so the utility of alternative data manipulations for a wide range of permeants remains to be validated.

2.5.2 Concentration Gradient or Thermodynamic Activity?

It was explained above that thermodynamic activity is the driving force for diffusion, but that concentration gradients are often used as an approximation, as they are easier to determine. The Fickian equations employ the concentration of permeant in the donor solution, assuming zero concentration in the receiving solution and so providing the maximal concentration gradient to drive drug transport. However, it is important to understand the thermodynamic drivers in transdermal and topical drug delivery.

Thermodynamic activity can be simplistically regarded as a measure of the "escape tendency" of a molecule from its solvent. By definition, a solid has a thermodynamic activity of 1, and so a saturated solution has a thermodynamic activity of 1, since any further molecules will generate a solid. Thus, a saturated solution has maximal thermodynamic activity and, equally, has the greatest concentration gradient across a membrane into a perfect sink containing no drug – hence their interchangeable use in the above equations (supersaturated states can have higher transient concentrations and thermodynamic activities and are discussed in Chapter 3). However, as concentration moves down from its saturation maxima, thermodynamic activity may not fall linearly.

Higuchi (1960) postulated that, when delivered from a vehicle that does not itself affect the skin membrane, then Equation 2.10:

$$J = \frac{DC_0}{h} \tag{2.10}$$

can be rewritten such that flux J (per unit area) can be described by:

$$J = \frac{D\alpha}{\gamma h} \tag{2.11}$$

where α is the thermodynamic activity of the drug in the vehicle, D is again the diffusion coefficient of the permeant, h remains the membrane thickness, and γ is the effective activity coefficient of the drug in the membrane. Analogous to the concentration term in Equation 2.10, Equation 2.11 shows that in order to obtain the maximum flux, the highest possible thermodynamic activity should be used.

Interestingly, and importantly for topical formulations, Higuchi's postulate also suggests that all vehicles (that don't interact with the skin membrane) containing a given drug at saturation will generate the same drug flux as they are all at the same, and maximal, thermodynamic activity. Though perhaps counterintuitive, the equation shows that a given drug delivered from a "good" solvent and saturated at 100 mg/mL would provide the same flux as when delivered from a poorer solvent, saturated at 1 mg/mL, assuming that the drug does not deplete significantly within the donor vehicle.

The important difference between concentration and thermodynamic activity was elegantly demonstrated by Theeuwes et al. (1976). Solutions of progesterone were prepared in water at 10 µg/mL and in polyethylene glycol at 2000 µg/mL. The solutions were separated by an inert polymer membrane and the redistribution of the drug assayed. Clearly, the concentration gradient in this case is from the highly loaded polyethylene glycol solution at 2000 µg/mL to the lower concentration aqueous solution at 10 µg/mL. However, as shown in Figure 2.4, drug transport was from the low concentration aqueous system into the higher concentration polyethylene glycol vehicle. This is because the aqueous solution at 10 µg/mL is near to saturation (solubility is 13.5 µg/mL, so it is at approximately 74% of solubility), and so is closer to maximal thermodynamic activity than when at 2000 µg/mL in polyethylene glycol (where solubility is 20,000 µg/mL, so it is at 10% of saturation, and far from its thermodynamic activity maxima). Equilibrium was reached when the concentration in the aqueous

Solubility in water = 13.5 µg/mL
Solubility in polyethylene glycol = 20,000 µg/mL

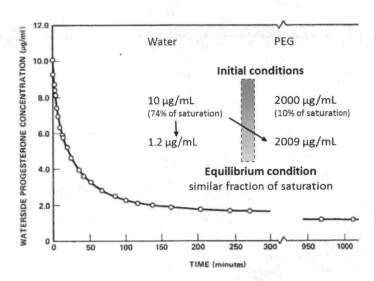

FIGURE 2.4 Progesterone flux across an ethylene-vinyl acetate copolymer membrane from a water solution at 10 µg/mL into a polyethylene glycol solution at 2000 µg/mL. (Modified from Theeuwes, F., Gale, R.M., and Baker, R.W, 1976. Transference: a comprehensive parameter governing permeation of solutes through membranes. *J. Membr. Sci.* 1: 3–16. With permission.)

phase fell to 1.2 µg/mL and rose in the polyethylene glycol phase to 2009 µg/mL; progesterone equilibrated to approximately 10% of solubility in each phase and were in thermodynamic activity equilibrium but clearly not at the same concentration.

2.5.3 Transient Permeation (Finite Dosing)

In most clinical situations, an infinite dose is not administered to a patient and in these circumstances of a finite dose application, pseudo steady-state permeation is unlikely to be achieved. In contrast to the infinite dose permeation profile shown in Figure 2.3, the cumulative permeation data when a finite dose has been applied increases to a plateau beyond which the amount permeated remains constant unless further doses are applied to the membrane surface (Figure 2.5). If the instantaneous flux values are plotted against time, then a peak in the profile is observed corresponding to the maximum flux that was delivered. Useful information can be gained from a cursory examination of instantaneous flux profiles from finite dose applications. For example, the breadth of the peak can indicate the extent of binding within the membrane, with broadly spread data suggesting that some of the dose is retained within the tissue for extended periods of time, possibly as a reservoir.

Applying a finite drug dose to skin membranes *in vitro* can be problematic, especially if using semi-solid formulations (detailed in Chapter 6). One approach is to apply a dilute solution in a volatile solvent that then evaporates from the tissue, leaving

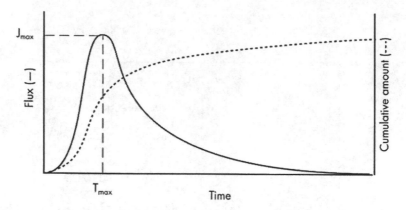

FIGURE 2.5 Typical permeation profile for a finite dose application to human skin membranes.

behind a thin film of the drug. This approach can raise questions as to the integrity of the membrane post-evaporation – are lipids removed from the stratum corneum by the solvent? – but since the process is usually rapid, then the risk of membrane damage is minimised. Advantageously, depositing the dose from a solvent helps the drug to be distributed evenly over the skin surface and can more easily deliver the required dose when compared to applying a semi-solid that is weighed and spread on the skin, since the solid material may be retained on the dosing or spreading implement.

With the finite dose protocol, several parameters tend to be reported from the instantaneous flux profiles. Generally reported are the maximum flux (J_{max}) and the time to maximum flux (T_{max}). It has been shown (Crank, 1975) that the magnitude of J_{max} is given by:

$$J_{max} = \frac{1.85 D C_0 \delta}{h^2} \tag{2.12}$$

where D is the apparent diffusion coefficient, C_0 is the concentration of the permeant in the first layer of the stratum corneum (this is maximal when the solid deposited drug is in contact with the skin surface), δ is the thickness of the finite dose layer on the skin surface, and h is the thickness of the stratum corneum. Similarly, the time to maximum flux can be represented by:

$$T_{max} = \frac{h^2 - \delta^2}{6D} \tag{2.13}$$

Since for a finite dose, δ must be considerably smaller than h, Equation 2.13 is usually approximated as:

$$T_{max} = \frac{h^2}{6D} \tag{2.14}$$

Thus, from both Equations 2.12 and 2.14, the apparent diffusion coefficient of the finite dose permeant can be estimated, accepting that many of the assumptions described above still apply.

The above intends to provide an introduction to simple mathematical treatments of skin permeation data. Far more sophisticated analyses are available and are described in the literature, building increasing complexity through compartmental approaches, defining diffusion parameters for each of the multiple pathways (intercellular, transcellular, and shunt routes), and including features such as binding and biotransformations. Alternative approaches are taken when, for example, assessing occupational risk of potentially hazardous materials. However, for most applications, the basic treatments above are suitable for assessing permeation data from relatively simple systems *in vitro*. Performance testing, including suitable design of *in vitro* permeation tests, is described in Chapter 6.

REFERENCES

Barbero, A.M. and Frasch, F. (2017). Effect of stratum corneum heterogeneity, anisotropy, asymmetry and follicular pathway on transdermal penetration. *J. Control. Release* 260: 234–246.

Barry, B.W. (1983). *Dermatological Formulations: Percutaneous Absorption*. New York, NY: Marcel Dekker Inc.

Bos, J. and Meinardi, M. (2000). The 500 Dalton rule for the skin penetration of chemical compounds and drugs. *Exp. Dermatol.* 9: 165–169.

Brown, M.B. and Jones, S.A. (2005). Hyaluronic acid: a unique topical vehicle for the localized delivery of drugs to the skin. *J. Eur. Acad. Dermatol. Venereol.* 19: 308–318.

Chen, M., Zakrewsky, M., Gupta, V., Anselmo, A.C., Slee, D.H., Muraski, J.A., and Mitragotri, S. (2014). Topical delivery of siRNA into skin using SPACE-peptide carriers. *J. Control. Release* 179: 33–41.

Crank, J. (1975). *The Mathematics of Diffusion*, 2nd edn. Oxford: Clarendon Press.

El Maghraby, G.M.M., Williams, A.C., and Barry, B.W. (2001). Skin hydration and possible shunt route penetration in controlled estradiol delivery from deformable and standard liposomes. *J. Pharm. Pharmacol.* 53: 1311–1322.

Essa, E.A., Bonner, M.C., and Barry, B.W. (2002). Human skin sandwich for assessing shunt route penetration during passive and iontophoretic drug and liposome delivery. *J. Pharm. Pharmacol.* 54: 1481–1490.

Essendoubi, M., Gobinet, C., Reynaud, R., Angiboust, J.F., Manfait, M., and Piot, O. (2016). Human skin penetration of hyaluronic acid of different molecular weights as probed by Raman spectroscopy. *Skin Res. Technol.* 22: 55–62.

Flynn, G.L. and Yalkowski, S.H. (1972). Correlation and prediction of mass transport across membranes. I. Influence of alkyl chain length on flux-determining properties of barrier and diffusant. *J. Pharm. Sci.* 61: 838–852.

Hedge, V., Hickerson, R.P., Nainamalai, S., Campbell, P.A., Smith, F.J., McLean, W.H., and Pedrioli, D.M. (2014). In vivo gene silencing following non-invasive siRNA delivery into the skin using a novel topical formulation. *J. Control. Release* 96: 355–362.

Higuchi, T. (1960). Physical chemical analysis of percutaneous absorption process from creams and ointments. *J. Soc. Cosmet. Chem.* 11: 85–97.

Hsu, T. and Mitragotri, S. (2011). Delivery of siRNA and other macromolecules into skin and cells using a peptide enhancer. *Proc. Natl. Acad. Sci.* 108: 15816–15821.

Lademann, J., Richter, H., Teichmann, A., Otberg, N., Blume-Peytavi, U., Luengo, J., Weiss, B., Schaefer, U.F., Lehr, C.M., Wepf, R., and Sterry, W. (2007). Nanoparticles – an efficient carrier for drug delivery into the hair follicles. *Eur. J. Pharm. Biopharm.* 66: 159–164.

Lauer, A.C., Ramachandran, C., Lieb, L.M., Niemiec, S., and Weiner, N.D. (1996). Targeted drug delivery to the pilosebaceous unit via liposomes. *Adv. Drug Deliv. Rev.* 18: 311–324.

Lenn, J., Neil, J., Donahue, C., Demock, K., Tibbetts, C.V., Cote-Sierra, J., Smith, S.H., Rubenstein, D., Therrien, J.-P., Pendergrast, S., Killough, J., Brown, M.B., and Williams, A.C. (2018). RNA aptamer delivery through intact human skin. *J. Invest. Dermatol.* 138: 282–290.

Mackay, K.M.B., Williams, A.C., and Barry, B.W. (2001). Effect of melting point of chiral terpenes on human stratum corneum uptake. *Int. J. Pharm.* 228: 89–97.

Miller, M.A., Yu, F., Kim, K.I., and Kasting, G.B. (2017). Uptake and desorption of hydrophilic compounds from human stratum corneum. *J. Control. Release* 261: 307–317.

Ossadnik, M., Czaika, V., Teichmann, A., Sterry, W., Tietz, H.J., Lademann, J., and Koch, S. (2007). Differential stripping: introduction of a method to show the penetration of topically applied antifungal substances into the hair follicles. *Mycoses* 50: 457–462.

Otberg, N., Richter, H., Schaefer, H., Blume-Peytavi, U., Sterry, W., and Lademann, J. (2004). Variations of hair follicle size and distribution in different body sites. *J. Invest. Dermatol.* 122: 14–19.

Roberts, M.S., Pugh, W.J., Hadgraft, J., and Watkinson, A.C. (1995). Epidermal permeability-penetrant structure relationships. 1. An analysis of methods of predicting penetration of monofunctional solutes from aqueous solutions. *Int. J. Pharm.* 126: 219–233.

Siddiqui, O., Roberts, M.S., and Polack, A.E. (1989). Percutaneous absorption of steroids: relative contribution of epidermal penetration and dermal clearance. *J. Pharmacokin. Biopharm.* 17: 405–424.

Sznitowska, M., Janicki, S., and Williams, A.C. (1998). Intracellular or intercellular localization of the polar pathway of penetration across stratum corneum. *J. Pharm. Sci.* 87: 1109–1114.

Taylor, N.A.S. and Machado-Moreira, C.A. (2013). Regional variations in transepidermal water loss, eccrine sweat gland density, sweat secretion rates and electrolyte composition in resting and exercising humans. *Extrem. Physiol. Med.* 2: 4.

Teichmann, A., Otberg, N., Jacobi, U., Sterry, W., and Lademann, J. (2005a). Follicular penetration: development of a method to block the follicles selectively against the penetration of topically applied substances. *Skin Pharmacol. Physiol.* 19: 216–223.

Teichmann, A., Jacobi, U., Ossadnik, M., Richter, H., Koch, S., Sterry, W., and Lademann, J. (2005b). Differential stripping: determination of the amount of topically applied substances penetrated into the hair follicles. *J. Gen. Intern. Med.* 20: 264–269.

Theeuwes, F., Gale, R.M., and Baker, R.W. (1976). Transference: a comprehensive parameter governing permeation of solutes through membranes. *J. Membr. Sci.* 1: 3–16.

Toll, R., Jacobi, U., Richter, H., Lademann, J., Schaefer, H., and Blume-Peytavi, U. (2004). Penetration profile of microspheres in follicular targeting of terminal hair follicles. *J. Invest. Dermatol.* 123: 168–176.

Touitou, E., Chow, D.D., and Lawter, J.R. (1994). Chiral beta-blockers for transdermal delivery. *Int. J. Pharm.* 104: 19–28.

Vickers, C.F. (1963). Existence of reservoir in the stratum corneum: experimental proof. *Arch. Dermatol.* 88: 20–23.

Williams, A.C. (2003). *Transdermal and Topical Drug Delivery.* London, UK: Pharmaceutical Press.

3 Chemical Modulation of Topical and Transdermal Permeation

3.1 INTRODUCTION

The range of drugs that can be delivered transdermally to therapeutic levels is restricted due to the effective barrier provided by skin, in particular the stratum corneum, as described in the earlier chapters. The magnitude of permeant flux was given by Equation 2.5 in Chapter 2 as:

$$\text{Flux} = \frac{\text{Diffusion coefficient} \times \text{partition coefficient} \times \text{concentration in the donor phase}}{\text{Membrane thickness}}$$

Various approaches have been used to modify the above parameters to increase drug flux: for example, the use of penetration enhancers or heat to increase drug diffusivity in the stratum corneum, application of prodrugs or solvents to change the formulation stratum corneum partition coefficient, and the use of supersaturated systems to increase the effective concentration in the applied formulation. Manipulating (reducing) skin thickness is difficult, though abrasion is widely used for callused skin, and the application site can be selected as one where the stratum corneum is relatively thin, such as the scrotum, which is used to deliver testosterone. Physical and technological approaches to enhance drug flux are described in Chapter 4, whereas this chapter considers chemical modulation of topical and transdermal permeation. Clearly there are opportunities to combine chemical and physical approaches, and these are summarised in Chapter 4 (Section 4.9).

3.2 CHEMICAL MODULATION OF DRUG FLUX

It has long been recognised that formulation components can influence transdermal and topical drug delivery. Over 40 years ago, Scheuplein (1977) reviewed work on the effects of solvents and surfactants on skin permeation and wrote:

> Skin permeability is increased by contact with a variety of liquids. Excluding highly corrosive chemicals, for example, concentrated acids and alkalis, there remain many substances which, although they do no great permanent damage, can markedly alter skin permeability.

The influence of stratum corneum hydration on drug permeation was initially demonstrated in a series of articles by Blank and co-workers (1952, 1953), Feldman

45

and Maibach (1965), and Scheuplein (1965). However, the first systematic reports of applying an exogenous chemical to enhance drug flux through human skin were in papers from Stoughton and Fritsch (1964), Horita and Weber (1964), and Jacob et al. (1964), using dimethyl sulphoxide (DMSO). Some 50 years later, DMSO is still being used in transdermal drug delivery studies and is an excipient in commercial products such as Pennsaid, a topical solution of 1.5% w/w diclofenac sodium containing >45% DMSO along with other solvents such as propylene glycol.

3.2.1 Mechanisms of Chemical Penetration Enhancement

Chemical penetration enhancers partition into, and interact with, stratum corneum components in a temporary and reversible manner. In comparison to physical enhancement techniques such as iontophoresis or electroporation, chemical permeation promoters are generally incorporated into "standard" formulations and so are amenable to existing manufacturing processes, and hence can be self-administered by patients. With a broad range of chemicals able to act as penetration enhancers, there is considerable design flexibility in their selection and use.

The mechanisms by which chemical penetration enhancers promote drug flux have been explored at various levels. Numerous structure–activity relationships have been developed for enhancers promoting different drug molecules, and these extend to consideration of the micro-environment provided by the enhancer at its site of action. The molecular interactions of enhancers with stratum corneum components (typically the multi-layered lipid domains) have been interrogated with increasingly sophisticated analytical techniques including small angle x-ray diffractometry and neutron scattering. Here, we consider enhancer actions in terms of the stratum corneum domains – the intercellular lipids, the corneocytes, and the influence on partitioning (Barry, 1991). A more detailed description of enhancer mechanisms of action and specific activities of chemicals that possess enhancement effects was recently provided by Dragicevic and Maibach (2015).

3.2.1.1 Interaction (Disordering) of Intercellular Lipids

Essentially, chemical penetration enhancers can disrupt the packing arrangement and organisation of the intercellular lipid bilayers of the stratum corneum. Other than shunt route delivery, permeants diffusing through the bulk of the stratum corneum must cross the intercellular lipid domains, irrespective of whether they also pass through or around the corneocytes. Thus, disruption of the intercellular lipids can promote drug delivery for permeants that predominantly exploit the intercellular or transcellular routes.

As described in Chapter 1 (Section 1.2.3.6), the stratum corneum lipid domains are heterogeneous with numerous packing motifs. Two lamella phases are seen, one with a short periodicity (repeat distance), and one with a longer repeat distance. The lateral organisation of the lipids is also complex. The orthorhombic phase dominates in healthy skin and has highly ordered and densely packed lipids that are essentially "crystalline" and so exhibit low permeability to drug molecules. Co-existing are the less densely packed, gel-like and more permeable hexagonal phase and the disordered, highly permeable liquid phase. Given this complexity, it is not surprising that,

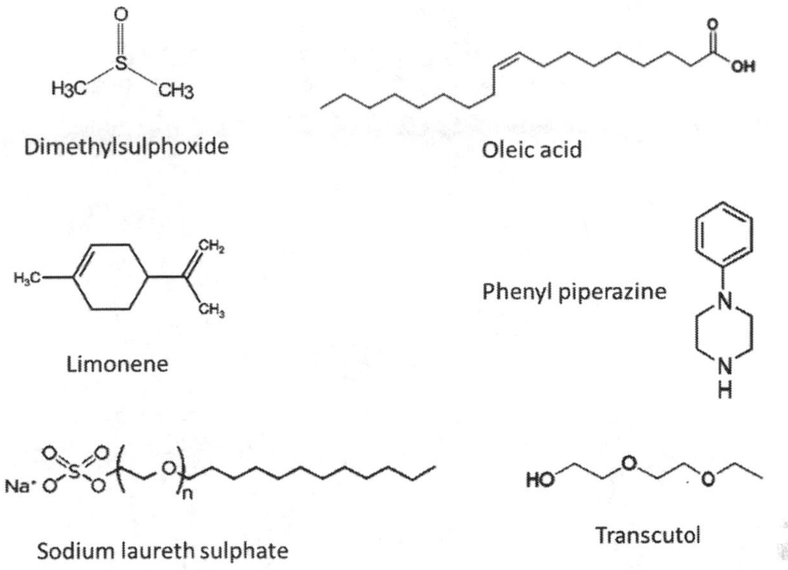

FIGURE 3.1 Examples to illustrate the varied structures of chemical penetration enhancers.

of the many enhancers that have some interaction with intercellular lipid bilayers, overarching comprehensive and predictive structure–activity relationships are lacking (Figure 3.1).

In general terms, materials with fatty chains appear to work well as intercellular lipid domain modifiers. For example, it could be anticipated that the acyl chains of oleic acid could insert into and intercalate with the intercellular lipid chains. Lipid chain length and the number of *cis*-double bonds appear to relate to fatty acid and fatty alcohol enhancement efficacies. For non-fatty enhancers such as DMSO or terpenes, which have also been shown to interact with the lipid domains, interaction with the intercellular lipid chains appears less likely, and these materials may preferentially distribute to the head groups of the lipid bilayers to distort the packing. Examples of potential interactions between some lipid-disrupting permeation enhancers and human stratum corneum bilayered lipids are illustrated in Figure 3.2.

3.2.1.2 Interactions within Corneocytes

Most research to develop and evaluate chemical penetration enhancers focusses on materials that perturb intercellular lipid domains, since these provide a barrier to either intercellular or transcellular drug transport. However, other excipients are known to exert some influence on the relatively dense corneocytes. In particular, keratolytic agents such as urea have been shown to enhance transdermal drug delivery, albeit (typically) to a lesser extent than agents which disrupt the lipid domains.

Given that the intercellular lipid domains provide the principal barrier to most drugs permeating through the stratum corneum, promoting diffusivity through the corneocytes per se is unlikely to have a major influence on drug delivery; perhaps some benefits accrue from the keratolytic agent in decreasing the thickness of the

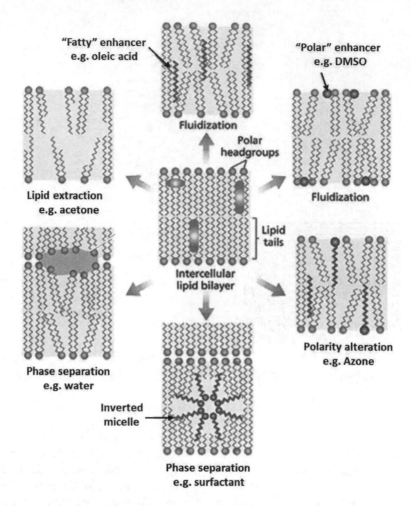

FIGURE 3.2 Potential interactions between chemical penetration enhancers and stratum corneum lipid domains. (Modified from Barry, B.W, 2004. Breaching the skin's barrier to drugs. *Nat. Biotechnol.* 22: 165–167. With permission.)

diffusional pathway, though again this is likely to be marginal. Thus, it is likely that enhancers acting on the corneocytes either directly or indirectly influence the intercellular lipid bilayers, or the covalently bound "anchor" lipids on the corneocyte membrane or perhaps split the desmosomes that provide adhesion between corneocytes. It should be borne in mind that chemical penetration enhancers within the skin are not restricted to a single simple mode of action. For example, urea is a keratolytic agent, but is also hygroscopic and can bind water, so it is a moisturising agent and could increase water content in the stratum corneum and, in addition, may also affect the lipid packing. Dimethyl sulphoxide can change the conformational state of keratin within the corneocytes, but also acts on lipid domains as described above. Anionic surfactants can uncoil keratin fibres, but also modify water binding within the tissue.

3.2.1.3   Alteration of Partitioning

Improving the partition coefficient of a drug between the applied vehicle and the stratum corneum generally improves delivery through the membrane; what goes in usually comes through, so increasing the amount of drug entering the stratum corneum typically improves flux. This can be achieved by altering the permeant – for example, with a prodrug, or using supersaturated systems (see below).

Improving the partitioning of a drug between the vehicle and the stratum corneum is thus a further mechanism of action described for chemical penetration enhancers. Solvents applied to the skin, and which diffuse well into the tissue, can act as a "sink" for drug partitioning; if a "good" solvent is included in the formulation, then, as the solvent itself permeates into the stratum corneum, drug solubility in the solvent within the tissue can increase. Such a reservoir effect has been shown for pyrrolidones, and also for commonly used formulation excipients such as propylene glycol. Of course, the solvent may also be useful for increasing the amount of another enhancer, such as oleic acid within the membrane, and highlights the importance of topical vehicle selection. Indeed, some standard "bases" for topical preparations contain significant quantities of enhancers, such as arachis oil which typically contains 35–72% oleic acid. Clearly, solvent diffusion from the stratum corneum (or clearance) can be more rapid than for the drug which can result in the drug becoming supersaturated within the stratum corneum and can lead to crystallisation (Hadgraft and Lane, 2016).

Selection of topical and transdermal formulation solvents clearly affects drug uptake into, and flux through, skin (Williams, 2007), but solvent supramolecular structuring has been used to promote drug residence in the epidermal tissue (Benaouda et al., 2016). By generating high concentrations of propylene glycol (PG) in the epidermis, diclofenac loading increased 175-fold compared to a control. At these high PG:water ratios, infrared studies showed supramolecular structures formed with strong physical affinity for the drug. Thus, a reservoir can be generated that could potentially offer sustained delivery from a topically applied formulation.

3.2.1.4   Other Mechanisms of Chemical Penetration Enhancement

The above mechanisms of action have been embraced within a general scheme to explain enhancer effects on stratum corneum, termed the lipid-protein-partitioning theory; enhancers can act by altering skin lipids and/or proteins and/or affecting partitioning behaviour (Barry, 1991). In addition to these three principal mechanisms of action, chemical penetration enhancers could operate directly or indirectly by:

1. Modification of thermodynamic activity of the vehicle. Rapid permeation of a good solvent from the donor solution, such as ethanol, can leave the permeant in a more thermodynamically active state than when the solvent was present – even to the point of supersaturation (see Section 3.4.4).
2. Solvent permeating through the membrane could "drag" the permeant with it.
3. Solubilisation of permeant in the donor – for example, by surfactants – especially where solubility is very low (as with steroids in aqueous donor solutions) can reduce depletion effects and prolong drug permeation.

4. Gross tissue damage: For example, high doses of potent solvents can damage the desmosomes responsible for cell adhesion, leading to fissuring of the intercellular lipid and splitting the stratum corneum layers. Also, high levels of solvent can partition into the corneocyte, disrupting the keratin, and can even form vacuoles. These effects are irreversible and so damage the tissue.
5. Metabolic manipulations: It is feasible that some chemicals interfere with the metabolic processes for the synthesis, assembly, activation, or processing of the intercellular lipid domains in the stratum corneum. This approach is problematic and is only included for completeness.

3.2.2 COMMON CHEMICAL PENETRATION ENHANCERS

An increasingly broad range of chemicals have been tested – or designed, synthesised, and tested – as penetration enhancers for transdermal drug delivery. Below are examples of materials that have been researched in some detail, with comments on their proposed mechanisms of action. Greater detail on individual chemical enhancers, reviewing their efficacies can be found in the chapters in Dragicevic and Maibach (2015).

To distinguish chemical penetration enhancers from other excipients, ideally an enhancer would:

- Have no pharmacological activity within the body
- Be non-toxic, non-irritating, and non-allergenic
- Work rapidly, and the scale of enhancement and its duration should be predictable and reproducible
- Have reversible action so that the skin barrier returns rapidly and fully
- Be suitable for formulation into topical preparations and so be compatible with drugs and excipients
- Be cosmetically acceptable with appropriate skin "feel"

3.2.2.1 Water

As noted above, the influence of occlusion (increasing the underlying water content of the stratum corneum) on drug permeation was reported in the 1950s, though earlier salves and balms probably exploited the occlusive effect. Water is thus the safest and most widely used chemical penetration enhancer and when used in typical formulations generally satisfies the above ideal characteristics for an enhancer, although prolonged occlusion can induce irritation.

The water content of human stratum corneum, under normal conditions is around 15 to 20% of the tissue dry weight (although this varies, depending on the external environment/humidity). Soaking in water, exposure to high humidities, or occlusion of the tissue reduces or prevents transepidermal water loss and hence increases the water content of the stratum corneum; following occlusion, the water content of the stratum corneum can increase to ~400% of the tissue dry weight. With such a highly complex heterogeneous structure as the stratum corneum, it is not surprising that the water contained within this membrane is found in several "states". Typically, from thermal analysis and spectroscopic methodologies, around 25–35% of the water present in stratum corneum can be described as "bound" (i.e., is associated with some structural element within the tissue). The remaining water can be considered "free" and is available to act as a solvent in the tissue. As described in Chapter 1 (Section 1.2.3.6), the stratum corneum contains Natural Moisturising Factor, a hygroscopic humectant mixture that retains water within the stratum corneum and maintains its pliability. Additionally, the keratin-filled corneocytes containing functional groups such as –OH and -COOH are expected to bind water molecules within the tissue. Considering these different water-binding sites, desorption of water from stratum corneum is complex. However, it is notable that even maintaining a stratum corneum membrane over a strong desiccant (e.g., phosphorous pentoxide) will not remove all the water from the tissue – there is a strongly bound fraction of around 5 to 10% that cannot be removed under such conditions.

The effectiveness of many topical preparations and products, such as patches and ointments, can be attributed (to a greater or lesser extent) to their occlusive effects which increases stratum corneum hydration to promote drug diffusivity through the membrane (see Chapter 5). Similarly, placing an occlusive dressing over the application site increases the hydration of the underlying stratum corneum and facilitates drug delivery. In general, increasing stratum corneum hydration tends to increase transdermal delivery of both hydrophilic and lipophilic permeants.

The precise mechanisms of action by which water increases transdermal drug flux are unclear. Free water within the tissue could alter the solubility of permeant in the stratum corneum and hence could modify partitioning of the agent from its vehicle into the membrane. Such a mechanism could partially explain elevated hydrophilic drug fluxes under occlusive conditions, but it does not explain hydration-enhanced delivery for lipophilic permeants, such as steroids, whose partitioning would be adversely affected.

The molecular dynamics in stratum corneum on heating and with hydration were studied by ^{13}C Solid-State NMR (Björklund et al., 2013). When relative humidity rose to 80–85%, a sharp change in keratin filament dynamics was observed. Interestingly, and in contrast to previous x-ray diffractometry studies, hydration was also shown to influence the intercellular lipids; at normal body temperature (32°C), the majority of the lipids are rigid (crystalline, orthorhombic) but co-exist with a small pool of mobile lipids (gel-like, hexagonal). The ratio between the mobile and rigid lipids increased with hydration and so can perhaps explain the hydration-induced increase in permeation of lipophilic drugs. Interestingly, heating the stratum corneum had a greater influence on lipid mobility, and mild heating has been used as an alternative (non-chemical) strategy to enhance transdermal drug delivery (see Chapter 4, Section 4.8).

3.2.2.2 Sulphoxides and Similar Chemicals

Dimethyl sulphoxide (DMSO) was one of the earliest and most widely studied penetration enhancers. It is a powerful aprotic solvent which can disrupt the hydrogen bonding network of water. It is colourless, odourless, and hygroscopic, and is often used in many areas of pharmaceutical sciences as a "universal solvent". DMSO alone has been applied topically to treat systemic inflammation, although presently it is used only to treat animals (e.g., horses, dogs).

The literature shows that DMSO is an effective penetration enhancer for both hydrophilic and lipophilic permeants and promotes transdermal permeation of, for example, antiviral agents, steroids and antibiotics. DMSO also works rapidly – spillage of the sulphoxide on the skin can be tasted in the mouth within seconds, most likely due to some shunt route transport. However, there are problems associated with DMSO whose effects are concentration dependent; relatively large proportions of this solvent are needed for significant enhancement. Further, at high concentrations, DMSO is irritant, causing erythema and wheals, and can also cause delamination of the stratum corneum whilst denaturing proteins. In addition, DMSO is metabolised via dimethyl sulphide which produces a foul odour to the breath. Thus, though the agent is a powerful and potentially valuable penetration enhancer, its use in commercial preparations is limited (Pennsaid is exceptional), and so researchers have sought other, chemically related, sulphoxide penetration enhancers (Figure 3.3).

Dimethylacetamide (DMAC) and dimethylformamide (DMF) are likewise powerful aprotic solvents with similar chemical structures to DMSO, though with nitrogen atoms rather than sulphur. Also, in common with DMSO, both these solvents have a broad range of penetration-enhancing activities, for example, promoting the flux of hydrocortisone, lidocaine, and naloxone through skin membranes. However, DMF may cause irreversible damage to the stratum corneum. Further structural analogues have been prepared including alkyl methyl sulphoxides such as decylmethyl sulphoxide (DCMS). This analogue has been shown to act reversibly on human skin and, like its parent DMSO, also possesses a concentration-dependent effect. DCMS appears to enhance hydrophilic permeants such as urea and 5-fluorouracil, but is less effective for promoting transdermal delivery of lipophilic drugs such as oestradiol.

The sulphoxides in general, and DMSO in particular, have varied mechanisms of action. DMSO is used in other fields as a cryoprotectant or to precipitate, crystallise, and denature proteins. It has been shown to change the intercellular keratin of

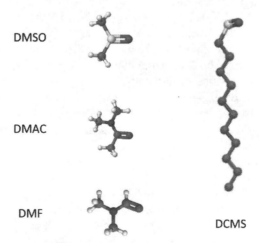

DMSO

DMAC

DMF

DCMS

FIGURE 3.3   Structure of some sulphoxides evaluated as chemical penetration enhancers. DMSO = dimethyl sulphoxide; DMAC = dimethylacetamide; DMF = dimethylformamide; DCMS = decylmethyl sulphoxide.

stratum corneum corneocytes from a predominantly α-helical to a β-sheet conformation. Studies also show that DMSO acts on the intercellular lipid domains, most
likely interacting with the polar heads group of some bilayer lipids to distort the
packing geometry of the barrier lipids.

3.2.2.3 Pyrrolidones

N-Methyl-2-pyrrolidone (NMP) and 2-pyrrolidone (2-P) are the most widely studied
enhancers of this group. NMP is a polar aprotic solvent and is used to extract aromatic moieties from oils, olefins, and animal feeds. It is a clear liquid at room temperature and is miscible with most common solvents, including water and alcohols.
Likewise, 2-P is miscible with many solvents, again including water and alcohols,
and is a liquid above 25°C. 2-pyrrolidone is also commonly used industrially and
is an intermediate in the manufacture of the widely used pharmaceutical excipient
polyvinylpyrrolidone. As with many penetration enhancers, the pyrrolidones tend to
show greater enhancement effects with hydrophilic permeants than with lipophilic
materials, although this may be attributable to the greater scope for enhancement of
inherently poorly permeating hydrophilic drugs.

When applied to skin, uptake of pyrrolidones into the tissue is high and so they effectively alter the solvent nature of the tissue; as strong solvents, they can increase drug
partitioning between the applied formulation and the skin, and solubilise the drug in
the stratum corneum. Thus, their prime mechanism of action appears to be the generation of a permeant reservoir within the tissue. The drug reservoir also offers potential
prolonged release of the permeant from the stratum corneum through to the systemic
circulation. However, clinical use of these enhancers is again precluded due to adverse
reactions. *In vivo* vasoconstrictor bioavailability studies have shown that pyrrolidones
cause erythema in some volunteers, although the effect was relatively short-lived.

3.2.2.4 Azone

Azone (1-dodecylazacycloheptan-2-one or laurocapram) was specifically designed as a
chemical penetration enhancer. It is a colourless, odourless liquid (melting point –7°C)
with a smooth, oily, but non-greasy feel. Its chemical structure (Figure 3.4) shows a
cyclic amide head group with an alkyl chain. As expected from its chemical structure,
it is a highly lipophilic material with a log $P_{octaol/water}$ around 6.2, and it is soluble in
and compatible with most organic solvents, including alcohols. The chemical has little
pharmacological activity, although some evidence exists for an antiviral effect, and it
has low toxicity (oral LD_{50} in rat of 9 g/Kg). Thus, Azone appears to possess many of
the desirable properties for the "ideal" penetration enhancer.

Azone is a potent and versatile enhancer for a range of drugs, and is effective for
both hydrophilic and lipophilic permeants. As with many penetration enhancers,
since permeation of lipophilic molecules tends to be relatively rapid, there may be
less scope to enhance the flux of lipophilic permeants than for hydrophilic molecules
where permeation is somewhat slower (Williams and Barry, 1991a). Thus, the most
dramatic flux improvements with Azone appear for permeants such as 5-fluorouracil
(flux enhanced ~100-fold through human epidermal membranes), with more moderate flux increases seen for lipophilic materials (betamethasone-17- benzoate flux
increased ~2-fold in man *in vivo*).

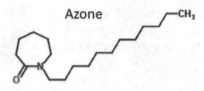

FIGURE 3.4   Chemical structure of Azone.

As with many chemical penetration enhancers, the effects of Azone are concentration-dependent, and efficacy is affected by the vehicle from which it is applied. The amount of Azone necessary to provide optimum enhancement varies between drugs and between formulations, but Azone is most effective at relatively low concentrations – typically less than 10% in the formulations, and often at around 1–3%. Propylene glycol has been shown to be an effective vehicle for delivering Azone to the stratum corneum, and indeed has been a valuable vehicle for delivering many enhancers to the skin.

Considering the chemical structure of the molecule, with a large polar head group attached to the alkyl chain, it is expected that the enhancer would distribute within the bilayered lipids to disrupt their packing arrangement. However, given the heterogeneity in stratum corneum lipid organisation, Azone is likewise expected to be present in various "domains" – interdigitated with stratum corneum lipids, and as "pools" or domains within the lipid bilayers. The "soup spoon" structure of Azone highlighted in Figure 3.4 illustrates how it would distort the stratum corneum intercellular lipids, and electron diffraction studies using lipids isolated from human stratum corneum provide good evidence that Azone exists (or partially exists) as a distinct phase within the stratum corneum lipids.

3.2.2.5   Fatty Acids

Numerous fatty acids have been tested and used as penetration enhancers. From the above examples, effective penetration enhancers such as Azone and decylmethylsulphoxide contain alkyl chains. Early structure–activity relationships showed that saturated C_{10} to C_{12} alkyl chains, attached to a polar head group, yielded potent enhancers, whereas with unsaturation in the alkyl chain, the C_{18} chain lengths appear near optimum (Aungst et al., 1986; Aungst, 1989).

Fatty acids have been used to enhance transdermal delivery of, amongst others, oestradiol, progesterone, acyclovir, 5-fluorouracil, retinoic acid, and salicylic acid and so are effective for both lipophilic and hydrophilic permeants (though again, flux of polar drugs appears to be improved to a greater extent than that of lipophilic permeants). Lauric acid (C_{12}) and stearic acid (IUPAC name octadecanoic acid, C_{18}) are potent straight chain fatty acid penetration enhancers whereas the *cis*-unsaturated oleic acid (C_{18}) is generally one of the prime enhancers selected for permeation investigations.

Considerable effort has been directed at investigating the mechanisms of action of fatty acids, and oleic acid in particular, as a penetration enhancer in human skin. As would be expected for a long chain fatty acid, it is apparent that these enhancers interact with the lipid domains within the stratum corneum. In addition, and

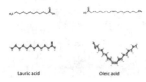

Lauric acid   Oleic acid

FIGURE 3.5 Chemical structure and 3D structure of the saturated fatty acid, lauric acid, and the unsaturated fatty acid, oleic acid.

similar to Azone, there is strong evidence that oleic acid exists in separate phases (or "pools") within the bilayer lipids. Whilst chemical structures are often drawn linearly, it is worth considering the three-dimensional structure of oleic acid. It is a mono-unsaturated omega-9 fatty acid, and so has a double bond at carbon number 9 (18:1 *cis*-9). In contrast to the saturated fatty acids, the molecule thus has a kink half-way along its alkyl chain. On insertion into an ordered lipid lamella, then the *cis* kink will increase the free volume present in the bilayer lipids, inducing significant disorder to the lipid bilayer packing, and this structural feature appears to be largely responsible for the potent enhancing effects seen with oleic acid (Figure 3.5).

3.2.2.6 Alcohols, Fatty Alcohols, and Glycols

Ethanol and other small alcohols such as propanol (isopropyl alcohol) are used in many transdermal and topical formulations, often as a solvent in the production of patches and in pharmaceutical and personal care (e.g., sunscreen) hydroalcoholic gels. As is the case with water, small alcohols such as ethanol permeate rapidly through human skin, with ethanol giving a steady-state flux of approximately 1 mg/cm^2/h. However, as a solvent, high concentrations of ethanol in the vehicle can extract lipids from stratum corneum membranes – and especially from more fragile animal tissue that may be used for *in vitro* permeation studies such as the hairless mouse.

Ethanol has been used to enhance the flux of both lipophilic and hydrophilic permeants but is more commonly employed with a co-solvent rather than neat. For ethanol/water co-solvent vehicles, the scale of penetration enhancement appears to be ethanol concentration-dependent; studies have shown that enhancement tends to increase to an optimal ethanol:water composition of ~0.63, above which enhancement effect declines. Ethanol is miscible in water and has complex concentration dependent behaviour in aqueous solutions. The alcohol (and other small alcohols such as methanol and propanol) forms strong hydrogen bonds with water molecules and ethanol–water networks have significant structuring. Clearly, the inclusion of a permeant into this network will distort the water–alcohol binding motif and influence delivery of the alcohol and permeant into the stratum corneum. Given that ethanol binds with water, then at higher ethanol concentrations, it is likely that the alcohol tends to dehydrate the stratum corneum which would inhibit permeation.

Ethanol enhances permeation through varied mechanisms. As a solvent, it can increase the solubility of the drug in a vehicle; although at steady state, the flux of a permeant from any saturated, non-enhancing, vehicle should be equivalent, increasing concentration of a poorly soluble drug can extend duration of steady-state drug delivery prior to depletion affecting flux. Additionally, permeation of ethanol into the stratum corneum can alter the solubility properties of the tissue with a consequent improvement of drug partitioning into the membrane. It is also feasible that the rapid permeation of ethanol, or evaporative loss of the solvent, from the donor phase modifies the thermodynamic activity of the drug in the formulation. This is most apparent when applying a finite dose of a drug onto the skin surface before evaporation of the ethanol; as the ethanol is lost, the drug concentration increases beyond its saturated solubility, providing a supersaturated state with a greater driving force for permeation (see Section 3.4.4). A further potential mechanism of action, arising as a consequence of rapid ethanol permeation across skin, is that a "solvent drag" effect may carry permeant into the tissue as the ethanol itself diffuses. Finally, when used at high concentrations for prolonged times, the solvent could extract stratum corneum lipids (though such an "enhancing" effect may be regarded as tissue damage, as it is not reversible).

Fatty alcohols (also termed "alkanols") are typically applied in a co-solvent (for example, propylene glycol), at between 1 and 10%. As with the fatty acids (Section 3.2.2.5), some structure/activity relationships for fatty alcohol penetration enhancement have shown lower activities for branched alkanols compared to linear molecules. For saturated fatty alcohols, efficacy tends to increase up to $\sim C_{10}$ and then falls as chain length increases further. As with the fatty acids, enhancement efficacy generally increases with the inclusion of up to two unsaturated bonds into the alcohols, again likely due to the formation of free volume within the intercellular lipid bilayers as the fatty alcohol intercalates into their structure. Oleyl alcohol (*cis*-9-octadecen-1-ol) is an unsaturated fatty alcohol that functions as a non-ionic surfactant and which has been widely used as a chemical penetration enhancer.

Glycols – notable propylene glycol and dipropylene glycol – have been used as a "stand-alone" penetration enhancer but are more widely used as vehicles with other chemical enhancers. Propylene glycol works synergistically with many enhancers, including Azone, oleic acid, fatty alcohols, and terpenes. These small glycols permeate well through human stratum corneum, and their mechanisms of action are probably similar to those suggested above for ethanol, but as relatively "mild" solvents, they are less likely to extract lipids from the stratum corneum. Permeation of the glycols themselves through the tissue could alter the composition, and hence the thermodynamic activity, of the drug in the remaining vehicle, which could in turn modify (increase) the driving force for drug diffusion. Uptake of the glycols into the stratum corneum could change the solvent properties of the tissue, thus facilitating uptake of the drug into skin, and there may be some minor disturbance to the intercellular lipid packing within the stratum corneum bilayers.

3.2.2.7 Surfactants

Surfactants are found in many existing therapeutic, cosmetic, and agrochemical preparations, and are clearly a major component of cleansing products (soaps, shampoos, etc.). Usually surfactants are added to formulations to solubilise lipophilic-active ingredients, and so they have potential to solubilise lipids within the stratum corneum. Generally composed of a lipophilic alkyl or aryl fatty chain, together with a hydrophilic head group, surfactants are often described in terms of their hydro-phile-lipophile balance (HLB). The HLB provides a measure of whether the surfactant is hydrophilic or lipophilic, drawn from the nature of the polar head group and hydrophobic fatty chain. The HLB value has thus been proposed as a means to predict penetration enhancement activity, but the literature shows that this is not a reliable tool, since the size and shape of the head and tail groups influence their enhancement activity.

Surfactants can be further classified according to the nature of the hydrophilic moiety; anionic surfactants have a negatively charged head group, such as from sulphate and phosphate moieties: for example, sodium lauryl sulphate (SLS). Cationic surfactants carry a positively charged head group that could be from a pH-dependent amine or from permanently charged quaternary ammonium salts, such as with cetrimonium bromide or benzalkonium chloride. Zwitterionic (amphoteric) surfactants have both cationic and anionic moieties attached to the same molecule, such as dodecyl betaine. Non-ionic surfactants are very commonly selected for use in transdermal and topical formulations and contain covalently bonded oxygen-containing hydrophilic head groups. There are many non-ionic surfactants available, including: poloxamers (triblock copolymers, known by their trade names Synperonics, Pluronics, and Kolliphor), sorbitan esters (also known as Spans), and polysorbates (known commonly as Tweens).

Anionic and cationic surfactants have the potential to damage human skin; SLS is a powerful irritant and increases the transepidermal water loss in human volunteers *in vivo*, and both anionic and cationic surfactants swell the stratum corneum and interact with the intercellular keratin. Non-ionic surfactants tend to be widely regarded as more acceptable for use in topically applied formulations, due to lower potential irritancy. Surfactants have generally low chronic toxicity, and most have been shown to enhance the flux of materials permeating through biological membranes.

As would be expected for charged materials, anionic and cationic surfactants tend to permeate relatively poorly though human stratum corneum when exposed for short time periods (i.e., when mimicking occupational exposure or washing), but permeation increases with application time. Likewise, the relatively large molecular weight of poloxamers, Tweens, and Spans also limit the permeation of non-ionic surfactants. However, surfactant-facilitated permeation of many materials through skin membranes has been researched. It appears that, in general terms, prolonged use of non-ionic surfactants has a minor enhancement effect in human skin, whereas anionic surfactants can have a more pronounced effect.

Surfactants can interact with skin constituents in various ways, depending on their nature. For example, they interact with proteins, can inactivate enzymes, and can bind within the stratum corneum. Anionic surfactants can swell the stratum corneum (probably by uncoiling the keratin fibres and altering the α-helices to a β-sheet conformation) and can modify the binding of water to the stratum corneum; anionic surfactant-treated stratum corneum is somewhat brittle, possibly due to the extraction of Natural Moisturising Factor. Harsh (typically charged) surfactants can also extract lipids from the stratum corneum, and can disrupt the lipid bilayer packing within the tissue. More generally, surfactants can modify the donor solution or formulation, altering the thermodynamics within the system to modify percutaneous drug delivery. However, with the problems of irritancy of anionic surfactants, and the low enhancement activity of non-ionic surfactants, these agents tend not to be used specifically as enhancers in topical formulation, though their presence may facilitate permeation.

3.2.2.8 Urea

Urea is a moisturising agent (a hydrotrope) used in the treatment of scaling conditions such as psoriasis, ichthyosis, and other hyperkeratotic skin conditions. Its structure allows each urea molecule to bind to five water molecules, and so it may hold water within the stratum corneum and thus facilitate transdermal permeation (since water is a potent enhancer itself). When used as a 10% cream, urea doubles the water-holding capacity of the stratum corneum, whilst having little effect on the transepidermal water loss, implying no damage to the tissue. Indeed, urea is also a component of endogenous Natural Moisturising Factor (Chapter 1, Section 1.2.6.3, and Figure 3.6).

Urea is also keratolytic, particularly after prolonged contact or when used at high concentrations, and has usually been used in combination with salicylic acid for keratolysis. The combination of increasing the water content of the stratum corneum with possible consequent effects on stratum corneum bilayer lipids together with modification to the intracellular keratin suggests that urea could be a potent penetration enhancer in human skin. However, the literature tends to show only modest enhancement effects of urea; to realise its keratolytic properties requires repeated application and the water bound to the urea molecule may not be available to act as an enhancer in the tissue. Rather than as a chemical penetration enhancer, urea is widely used as an emollient in many topically applied formulations.

Modified urea analogues have been synthesised in attempts to combine the water holding and keratolytic properties of urea with moieties that have shown enhancement

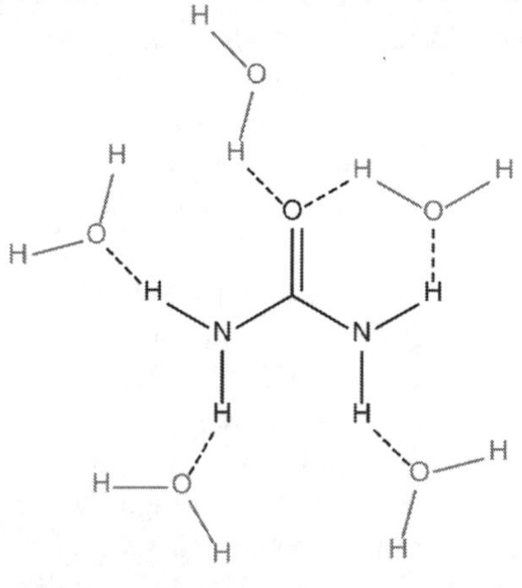

FIGURE 3.6   Structure of urea the structure of urea with five water molecules coordinated.

activity (such as C_{12} alkyl chains). For example, a series of C_{12} alkyl- and aryl-substi-tuted urea analogues were moderately effective as enhancers for 5-fluorouracil when applied in propylene glycol to human skin *in vitro*, though urea itself was ineffective (Williams and Barry, 1989).

3.2.2.9   Terpenes

Terpenes, and their parent essential oils, have long been used as medicines, flavour-ings, and fragrance agents. For example, menthol is traditionally inhaled for con-gestion and sinus problems, and it has a mild antipruritic effect when incorporated into emollient preparations. It is also used as a fragrance and to flavour toothpastes, peppermint sweets, and mentholated cigarettes.

Terpenes contain only carbon, hydrogen, and oxygen atoms but are not aromatic. They are based upon isoprene units (C_5H_8) and are classified by their chemical struc-ture, so that monoterpenes (C_{10}) contain two isoprene units, sesquiterpenes (C_{15}) have three, diterpenes (C_{20}) have four isoprene units, and so on. Further, terpenes may be acyclic or cyclic (mono-cyclic, bi-cyclic, etc.), and are found with varied function-alities such as hydrocarbons, alcohols, ketones, and oxides. Given their widespread availability and broad range of structural features, numerous terpenes (and their par-ent essential oils) have been evaluated as chemical penetration enhancers.

Early work sought to elucidate structure–activity relationships for a broad range of monoterpenes (Williams and Barry, 1991a,b). In general, hydrocarbon terpenes such as d-limonene were potent enhancers for lipophilic permeants, whereas terpenes with an electro-negative oxygen atom, such as the ketones pulegone or carvone, and oxides such as 1,8-cineole were potent enhancers for a hydrophilic drug (5-fluoro-uracil). This is perhaps not surprising since the terpenes tend to be relatively "good" solvents and are readily taken up into the stratum corneum where they could then promote uptake of the permeant into the tissue. When applied from a co-solvent, such as propylene glycol, terpene uptake and enhancement potency also seem to be elevated. As with many of the other chemical penetration enhancers described above, loss of a terpene from a formulation (due to either evaporation or permeation into the skin) can alter the thermodynamic activity of the drug in the formulation, which could elevate drug flux. Terpenes also modify drug diffusivity through the membrane; a reduction in the lag time for permeation is usually found, indicative of increased drug diffusivity through the membrane (see Chapter 2, Section 2.4). Small angle x-ray diffraction studies have indicated that d-limonene and 1,8-cineole disrupt stratum corneum bilayer lipids whereas nerolidol, a long chain sesquiterpene reinforces the bilayers, possibly by orientating alongside the stratum corneum lipids. Spectroscopic evidence has also suggested that, as with Azone and oleic acid, terpenes could exist within separate domains in stratum corneum lipids.

3.2.2.10   Phospholipids

Many studies have employed phospholipids as vesicles (liposomes) to carry drugs into and through human skin and they have been suggested as penetration enhancers in a non-vesicular form. Considering their physicochemical properties and struc-tures, it may be expected that phospholipids would interact with the bilayer lipids of the stratum corneum to disrupt their packing geometry. However, there is no compelling evidence to suggest that phospholipids interact directly with stratum corneum lipids. This may be due to the difficulty in delivering these typically large molecules through the stratum corneum, or perhaps that they are unable to integrate with the bilayer lipids within the stratum corneum – which do not contain endogenous phospholipids (Chapter 1, Section 1.2.3.6). However, phospholipids can occlude the skin surface, and thus can increase tissue hydration which, as shown above, can increase drug permeation. When applied to the stratum corneum as vesicles, phospholipids can fuse with stratum corneum lipids. This structural collapse liberates the permeant into a dynamically changing vehicle in which the drug is usually poorly soluble, and hence thermodynamic activity is raised so can promote drug flux.

3.2.2.11 Amino Acid–Based Enhancers

Amino acids comprise ~40% of Natural Moisturising Factor, of which L-serine is the most abundant (~36%), followed by glycine (22%) and L-alanine (13%). Interestingly, these natural amino acids are frequently associated with water-retentive properties not only in skin but also, for example, in atmospheric aerosols and silks.

A series of amino acid derivatives were synthesised in attempts to enhance the water-holding capacity of the natural parent amino acid (Arezki et al., 2017). Thus, analogues with increasing levels of the electronegative oxygen atom were developed and were shown to bind greater numbers of water molecules compared to the parent amino acid; for example, each N-hydroxyserine bound to 12 water molecules (by thermal analysis and molecular modelling), whereas each L or D-serine molecule bound 0.5 water molecules (Figure 3.7).

Other analogues of amino acids have been developed, including the addition of alkyl chains. For example, DDAIP (N,N-dimethylalanine dodecyl ester) is an amphiphilic molecule with a pKa of 4.87 and which has high water solubility (Figure 3.8). Interestingly, the molecule is an ester of N,N-dimethylalanine and dodecanol; the C_{10} fatty alcohols were shown above to have greatest enhancement activity of this class of molecules (Section 3.2.2.6). DDAIP is one of few molecules designed and used as a chemical penetration enhancer. As an ester, it is readily metabolised on and in the skin to liberate N,N-dimethylalanine which is further metabolised to alanine, an

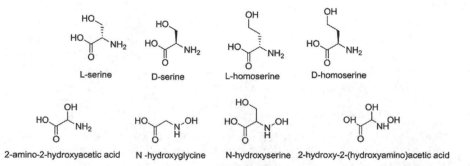

FIGURE 3.7 Structure of some modified hygroscopic linear amino acids designed to increase water-holding capacity in stratum corneum.

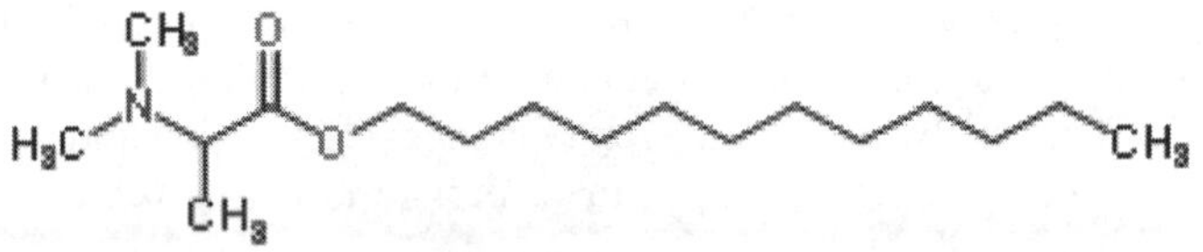

FIGURE 3.8 Chemical structure of DDAIP, an ester of N,N-dimethylalanine and dodecanol.

endogenous amino acid, and dodecanol, which is oxidised to another endogenous material, lauric acid. Given its chemical structure, it is apparent that the molecule would be expected to interact with the stratum corneum bilayer lipid organisation to promote drug diffusivity, and may also impact drug uptake into the tissue.

3.2.2.12 Peptides

Numerous peptides have been evaluated as penetration enhancers in human skin. These have included cell-penetrating peptides, membrane-penetrating peptides (such as antimicrobial peptides) and phage peptides. Studies have evaluated the enhancement effects of the peptides alone, or when they are used as a conjugate to carry a drug cargo, for both small and relatively large molecular weight drugs.

Cell-penetrating peptides were first reported in 1988 when it was found that the Trans-Activator of Transcription (TAT) protein from the human immunodeficiency virus 1 (HIV-1) entered tissue-cultured cells and promoted viral gene expression. Subsequently, numerous peptides showing similar cell-penetrating capacities have been discovered or, in some cases, rationally designed. Typically, cell-penetrating peptides are relatively short (up to ~30 residues) and can cross varied cell membranes with little or no toxicity using energy-dependent and/or independent mechanisms. Commonly, they carry multiple positively charged amino acids such as arginine or lysine – often termed polycationic – or have a sequence of alternating charged and non-polar amino acids.

Intuitively, it would not be expected that charged molecules with a molecular weight up to ~3000 Da would enter the stratum corneum. Nonetheless, the literature contains reports of enhanced topical delivery of small drug molecules, siRNA, proteins, peptides, and nanoparticles by cell-penetrating peptides, most commonly as a conjugated system. Whilst some studies employ human skin, many reports describe delivery enhanced in animal tissue, notably hairless mouse skin, which is considerably more fragile than human skin, and so such results should be viewed with some caution.

Membrane-penetrating peptides also tend to carry a positive charge, but may be between 12 and 100 amino acids. As antimicrobial peptides, they play a significant role in host defence against microbial assault, since they depolarise membranes and so disrupt membrane lipids (hence their purported value as skin penetration enhancers).

3.2.3 Synergy between Chemical Penetration Enhancers

It is apparent from the above that many penetration enhancers appear to be most effective when used in combination – for example, employing oleic acid in combination

with propylene glycol. This may help to exploit thermodynamic principles by optimising the delivery of one (or more) enhancer in a formulation, or it may exploit
the varied mechanisms by which different enhancer exert their effects. Combining
enhancers thus provides greater scope to formulate effective vehicles to enhance
drug delivery.

When combining chemical penetration enhancers, their efficacy can simply be
additive; if the flux of a drug increases by a factor of 2 by one enhancer and a factor
of 3 by another, an additive effect would increase flux by a factor of 5. Synergy is
seen when the combination enhances drug flux to a greater (or indeed, lesser) extent
than when the enhancers work independently. Thus, positive synergy in the above
example would occur when flux is increased greater than 5-fold – and negative synergy when the flux increase was less than a factor of 5.

Synergistic combinations of penetration enhancers are difficult to predict for
any particular permeant, and so synergy has often been discovered serendipitously
through experimentation. Most notably, synergy is often reported when an anticipated
chemical penetration enhancer, such as Azone or oleic acid, is applied in a solvent
which itself may have some very limited enhancement efficacy, such as propylene glycol. Beyond Azone and oleic acid, synergy has been reported when various terpenes
are used in propylene glycol, between dimethyl sulphoxide and propylene glycol when
used as a vehicle, and when urea and analogues were delivered from propylene glycol.
Synergy has also been reported between ethanol and various enhancers, and for other
solvents such as dimethylisosorbide, with enhancers including fatty acids.

However, there have been impressive attempts made to screen relatively large
libraries of enhancer combinations. For example, an IN-vitro Skin Impedance-
Guided High-Throughput (INSIGHT) screening method was used to assess the
potency of penetration enhancer mixtures in an array format (Karande et al., 2004).
Using electrical conductivity across the skin as a surrogate measure of skin permeability, the method allowed a library of over 5000 penetration enhancer mixtures
to be screened. Interestingly, of these, only ~2% were shown to act synergistically.
Positive hits from the screen were then validated by skin permeation experiments
using Franz diffusion cells. It was notable that two of the most potent enhancer combinations were sodium lauryl ether sulphate with 1-phenylpiperazine, and N-lauroyl
sarcosine with sorbitan monolaurate (Karande et al., 2007). Other than the pipera-
zine, the other three enhancers are surfactants and are not widely regarded as potent
enhancers on their own.

3.2.4 General Comments on Penetration Enhancers

The above descriptions of chemicals that have been used as penetration enhancers is clearly not exhaustive but illustrates the broad range of agents that have been
employed to facilitate topical and transdermal drug delivery. Clearly it is feasible to
promote transdermal delivery of both hydrophilic and hydrophobic small molecule
drugs and the rational design of synergistic enhancer combinations or use of peptides
may allow delivery of larger therapeutic molecules into human skin.

Chemicals with penetration-enhancing activity are already well-accepted in
numerous formulations, both for topical and transdermal delivery. For example,

olive oil contains high levels of the well-established penetration enhancer oleic acid, alongside significant amounts of other enhancing chemicals such as linoleic acid and palmitic acid. Ethanol and propylene glycol are commonly used in patches, surfactants stabilise creams, ethanol is a significant component of many hydroalcoholic gels, and terpenes are often selected as fragrance agents. However, penetration enhancement by these excipients is often coincidental to their main functions as vehicles, solvents, and stabilisers. The widespread use of these enhancing excipients gives some confidence of their safety profiles, though clearly local irritation and adverse reactions will depend on excipient concentration and release (delivery) from a given formulation during its period of use – which can vary from a short-term application of a hydroalcoholic gel to 7-day wear of a transdermal patch. As a caveat, it should also be noted that many novel penetration enhancers are investigated using *in vitro* testing protocols, and may not be suitable for *in vivo* application – perhaps due to adverse skin reactions or incompatibilities (physical and/or chemical) with other excipients. The FDA provides an Inactive Ingredient Database that shows whether an excipient has previously been used in an FDA-approved product and can be a useful source for selecting potential enhancers.

Several common themes can be drawn for chemical penetration enhancers:

- Penetration enhancers tend to work well with co-solvents such as propylene glycol or ethanol. Synergistic effects are found between enhancers such as Azone, oleic acid (and other fatty acids), and terpenes with propylene glycol.
- Most penetration enhancers have complex concentration-dependent effects, especially when used with co-solvents, such as ethanol or propylene glycol.
- Potential mechanisms of action of enhancers are varied and can range from direct effects on the skin to modification of the formulation. Most enhancers operate through a combination of mechanisms which can include:
  a. Acting on the stratum corneum intracellular keratin to denature or modify its conformation, causing swelling and increased hydration/ plasticisation.
  b. Affecting the desmosomes that maintain cohesion between corneocytes.
  c. Modifying the intercellular lipid domains to reduce the barrier resistance of the bilayer lipids. Disruption to the lipid bilayers could be homogeneous where the enhancer distributes evenly within the complex bilayer lipids, but it is more likely the enhancer will be heterogeneously distributed within domains of the bilayer lipids, forming "pools".
  d. Altering the solvent nature of the stratum corneum to increase uptake of the drug or of a co-solvent into the tissue. Most enhancers are good solvents for the permeating drug molecule and so can increase the amount of permeant present within the skin, essentially forming a drug reservoir in the tissue.
  e. Modification of the thermodynamic activity of the drug in its residual vehicle. Rapid permeation of a good solvent from the donor solution, such as ethanol, can leave the permeant in a more thermodynamically active state than when the solvent was present – even to the point of supersaturation (see Section 3.4.4).

    f. Solvent permeating through the membrane could "drag" the permeant with it.

    g. Solubilisation of the permeant in the donor (e.g., with surfactants), especially where solubility is very low, for example, as with steroids in aqueous donor solutions, can reduce depletion effects and prolong drug permeation.

It should also be noted that there remain some issues and areas of concern when using chemical penetration enhancers. In particular:

- Rationally selecting a penetration enhancer for a given permeant is problematic. Enhancer potencies are difficult to predict and so selecting an enhancer for a particular drug is difficult. There are some general trends whereby, for example, hydrocarbon monoterpenes tend to enhance delivery lipophilic permeants, but the level of enhancement is unpredictable.
- There are significant inter-species differences in penetration enhancer potencies, and efficacies in animal skins, and rodent skins in particular, are generally considerably greater than those obtained with human skin. Caution should be used when extrapolating data showing enhancement of drug delivery using, for example, hairless mouse skin, to human skin.
- Though "safe" enhancers have been described in the literature, and materials are claimed to be non-irritating, it is conceptually difficult to see how any chemical that disrupts the normal stratum corneum barrier layer (lipids, proteins, desmosomes, etc.) can have no adverse effects. Indeed, in order to enhance transdermal drug delivery, it is intuitive that some disruption of skin homeostasis is necessary. Thus, enhancers may have low or acceptable risks associated with them, but even the most "inert" of enhancers, water, can adversely affect skin structure. Naturally, the risks should be correlated with clinical benefits and with the adverse effects associated with alternative routes of drug delivery, such as hepatic metabolism and consequent side effects or adverse effects on gastrointestinal epithelia.
- Many, if not most, enhancers act by multiple mechanisms in the stratum corneum, and when accelerants are combined to produce synergistic enhancement, then the mechanisms operating become even more complex. It is thus difficult to provide conclusive proof that a simple mechanism of action operates which can cause regulatory unease.

3.3 PERMEATION RETARDATION

Given the remarkable barrier properties of human skin, and that the stratum corneum limits drug administration, pharmaceutical formulators generally focus on strategies to enhance topical and transdermal drug delivery. However, inhibition or retardation of topical and transdermal permeation can be useful in other sectors such as agrochemicals and for some personal care products.

Various strategies can be employed to reduce transdermal permeation of undesirable materials, essentially reversing the principles outlined above and below to maximise drug delivery. For example, a formulation can be modified to minimise the thermodynamic activity of the agent in its vehicle and hence limit permeant entry into the stratum corneum. Permeation can also be retarded by the use of barrier creams, some chemicals have been shown to act as chemical penetration retarders, and formulation excipients can be included to minimise permeant flux.

Personal protective equipment (PPE), such as protective gloves, provides a physical barrier that prevents skin exposure to an unwanted permeant. Whilst clearly appropriate in many situations, there are many reports that the use of inappropriate clothing can exacerbate percutaneous absorption of toxic agents. For example, it is conceivable that a highly lipophilic pesticide could partition well into a lipophilic glove to form a reservoir of the pesticide that could permeate the skin over an extended time frame. Where gloves are not appropriate or are restrictive for performing required operations, an alternative approach can be to use a barrier cream.

Barrier creams vary from a simple application of petroleum jelly to more elegant formulations. When selecting a barrier cream, it is important to understand the nature of the permeant against which protection is sought, and there are numerous examples in the literature where an inappropriate barrier cream has been ineffective or, worse, delivered the undesired permeant. For example, an *in vivo* study of three barrier creams protecting against hydrophilic and lipophilic dyes showed that one cream did decrease the amounts of both dyes in the skin samples, another formulation protected against the lipophilic dye but not against the hydrophilic permeant, whereas the third cream formulation *increased* the levels of both dyes within the tissue (Zhai and Maibach, 1996). Barrier creams tend to be designed to protect against lipophilic permeants such as pesticides and herbicides (since permeation of hydrophilic permeants is inherently relatively low). Barrier preparations are themselves typically lipophilic in order to capture and "trap" the lipophilic agents. However, as occlusive coverings to the skin surface, lipophilic barrier creams can dramatically increase the water content of the stratum corneum, with consequent potential for increased permeant flux as described above.

Permeation retarders are materials with the opposite effect to enhancers – they interact with skin components to decrease flux. Such materials could act by modification of the intracellular keratin, by altering partitioning into the tissue (i.e., by using an antisolvent), or by increasing the "rigidity" or barrier nature of the stratum corneum lipids. This last approach, to increase the order of lipid bilayers within the stratum corneum by adding further lipid like molecules, though intuitively unlikely, has shown promise. An analogue of Azone, N-0915, reduced the flux of both metronidazole and the insect repellent diethyl m-toluamide (DEET) though human epidermal membranes, whereas Azone enhanced fluxes (Hadgraft et al., 1996). These opposing properties of the two analogues probably result from their chemical structures; Azone adopts a soup spoon structure providing a larger area per molecule (illustrated in Section 3.2.2.4), whereas N-0195 is more linear and with a charge distribution that may favour electrostatic interactions with stratum corneum lipids.

Cyclodextrins are host molecules that form inclusion complexes in both solid and solution phases. The cavity within these cyclic sugars is hydrophobic and hence lipophilic guest molecules that fit, at least partially, into the cavity can form relatively stable complexes. The exterior of the sugar is hydrophilic and so a cyclodextrin/lipophilic guest complex tends to increase the apparent aqueous solubility of the guest.

Cyclodextrins are also relatively large molecules, typically >1000 Da and so would be expected to traverse human skin poorly.

The benefits and limitations of cyclodextrin use in transdermal drug delivery remain controversial. Some reports show that they increase drug flux, notably in animal tissue, and they may extract some lipids from the stratum corneum. In contrast, others reported that cyclodextrins do not enhance drug flux through interaction with skin components, but that increased delivery for some materials could be explained by the solubilising effect of the sugars on drugs in donor solutions. Further, excess of the complexing host molecules in a formulation can reduce the flux of a permeant by essentially forming a large molecular weight complex that limits drug presence at the skin surface. Various cyclodextrins formed host:guest inclusion complexes with the lipophilic permeant oestradiol, and reduced flux through human skin, but, as expected, had no effect on flux of the non-complexing hydrophilic guest 5-fluorouracil; further, cyclodextrins in a protective ointment base retarded toluene permeation through human skin membranes (Williams et al., 1998).

3.4 DRUG AND FORMULATION MANIPULATION STRATEGIES

Beyond the use of chemical penetration enhancers directly acting on the stratum corneum, alternative strategies can be used to manipulate transdermal drug delivery. The physicochemical nature of the permeant can be altered to provide a drug form with improved partitioning/permeation characteristics; the prodrug so formed is later cleaved within the body to liberate the active molecule. Other manipulations to improve drug delivery can be carried out by forming ion-pairs between a charged permeant and an excipient, forming eutectic systems, or by manipulating the formulation to generate supersaturated systems.

3.4.1 PRODRUGS

An early and widely adopted strategy to optimise both local and systemic delivery of topically applied agents has been the use of prodrugs. As described in Chapter 2 (Section 2.5.1, Equation 2.5), the steady-state flux of a permeant through skin is proportional to the partition coefficient of the permeant between the stratum corneum and the donor formulation.

If the permeant does not possess the appropriate physicochemical properties to enter the stratum corneum from the vehicle, then one option is to design a prodrug with more suitable attributes for topical and transdermal drug delivery. Naturally, changing the nature of the permeant will also affect its solubility in a given vehicle and its diffusion coefficient in the membrane, both of which are also directly proportional to the drug flux.

Generally, prodrugs for topical application are designed with lipophilic moieties attached to the parent compound, since the increased lipophilicity facilitates partitioning of the permeant into the stratum corneum. Once in the tissue, the prodrug may be stable to enzymatic conversion within the viable epidermis and so pass intact through to the systemic circulation for activation, or the prodrug may be cleaved in the skin to liberate the active compound. The skin contains appreciable non-specific esterase activity, and this has been exploited for delivering a wide range of ester-based prodrugs.

The clearest illustration of the value of prodrug development is seen with topical corticosteroids. As a valerate (C_4H_9COOH) ester, betamethasone valerate 0.05% ointment is classed as moderately potent (UK Class III, U.S. Class 4/5). However, betamethasone dipropionate 0.05% ointment is classed as highly potent (UK Class II, U.S. Class 2/3) and when in an optimised ointment formulation, the same concentration of the dipropionate ester is classed as super potent (UK Class I, U.S. Class 1). The selection of the prodrug moiety affects uptake of the drug into the skin, as well as the rate of de-esterification and clinical efficacy. Other commonly used prodrug moieties for steroids include acetate (e.g., hydrocortisone acetate, low potency), acetonide (e.g., triamcinolone acetonide, moderate potency) and furoate (e.g., mometasone furoate, high potency).

Beyond steroid esters, prodrugs for topical dosing have been developed and evaluated for wide-ranging pharmaceutical actives, including:

- Anti-retrovirals, such as methoxypolyethylene glycol carbonate derivatives of zidovudine.
- Non-steroidal anti-inflammatory agents, for example, piperazinylalkyl ester prodrugs and polyoxyethylene glycol ester prodrugs of ketorolac; ethylene glycol, glycerol, and 1,3-propylene glycol esters of diclofenac.
- Opioid analgesics, such as morphine propionate and morphine enanthate.
- Opioid antagonists, for example, naltrexone with straight- and branched-chain alkyl ester.
- Anti-parkinsonian drugs, such as the diesters diacetyl apomorphine and diisobutyryl apomorphine.
- Anti-schizophrenic agents, such as ethyl, propyl, butyl, octyl, and decyl esters of haloperidol.
- Anti-cancer agents. For example, 5-aminolevulinic acid (5-ALA) is a prodrug used in photodynamic therapy to treat skin cancers. The prodrug converts to protoporphyrin IX, which is an effective photosensitiser, via the heme biosynthetic pathway. However, 5-ALA is inherently unstable, and permeates the skin poorly; attempts have been made to enhance permeation of this molecule using alternative prodrugs that are more lipophilic.

As described earlier, many enhancement strategies can be used synergistically, for example, combining an appropriate co-solvent with a penetration enhancer. Similarly, some prodrugs have been designed to possess an established enhancing moiety. Thus, alkylazacycloalkan-2-one esters of indomethacin have been synthesised, and fatty acid ester derivatives of cycloserine tested.

3.4.2 ION-PAIRING

Given that the principal barrier to topical and transdermal drug delivery results from the stratum corneum intercellular lipid domains, charged (hydrophilic) species do not readily partition into, or permeate through, human skin membranes. One approach to overcome this limitation is to form an ion-pair by combining an oppositely charged species with the charged permeant; theoretically, a complex is formed in which the charges are neutralised. Unlike a prodrug with a covalent bond between the active agent and the lipophilic moiety, ion-pairs form through electrostatic interactions. With the charges effectively neutralised, the ion-pair more readily enters the stratum corneum where it may then dissociate to liberate the charged species.

Counter ions can directly influence the effective physicochemical properties of the parent drug, such as lipophilicity. Ion-pairing can be simply through the selection of a salt for the active drug, such as the use of the sulphate of terbutaline or lignocaine hydrochloride. Alternatively, counter ions can be selected to possess chemical penetration-enhancing activity. For example, oleic acid was paired with ondansetron, salicylates have been paired with amines and quaternary ammonium ions, and ion-pairs of loxoprofen with organic amines such as trimethylamine have been shown to enhance flux of this non-steroidal anti-inflammatory agent.

Ion-pairing and the effects on permeation can be complex. Investigating permeation of propranolol through human skin, Stott et al. (2001) found that the β-blocker formed a 1:1 addition compound with several fatty acids. Infrared spectral studies showed that, for example, lauric acid and propranolol permeate at a rate equivalent to a 1:1 mole ratio through human skin membranes when applied concurrently, consistent with the two species permeating via an ion-pairing mechanism. However, as with many other studies, the scale of enhancement from ion-pairing appears relatively small, with doubling of drug fluxes typically reported. More recently, a mechanistic study explored delivery of bisoprolol from ion-pairs with a homologous series of saturated fatty acids (C_6 to C_{18}) (Zhao et al., 2017). By selecting a homologous series of counter ions, factors such as the complex's polar surface area, stability, and physicochemical properties were controlled. From *in vitro* permeation studies through rat skin, the permeability coefficient of bisoprolol itself was 1.9×10^{-3} cm/h. As an ion-pair with the fatty acids, permeability coefficient generally increased with a maximal value for the C_6 (hexanoic acid) counter ion of 22.6×10^{-3} cm/h. The permeants were applied to the skin as suspensions (hence saturated). As the ion-pair is more lipophilic than the charged drug, solubility in the donor vehicle fell with ion-paring. Since flux is the product of permeability coefficient and applied (effective) concentration, these differences in solubility impacted delivery of the drug. Consequently, the flux of bisoprolol alone was 250 µg/cm²/h, whereas the hexanoic acid ion-pair flux was only 212 µg/cm²/h, and this fell with the longer chain fatty acids down to 40 µg/cm²/h for the C_{18} counter ion. The authors also noted that the ion-pairs survived within the stratum corneum, but dissociated in the viable epidermal layer, and that this may play a controlling role in bisoprolol delivery.

Coacervation is a somewhat specialised form of ion-pairing and is usually used to describe electrostatically driven liquid–liquid phase separation when oppositely charged macromolecular ions associate; one liquid phase is a concentrated colloidal phase (the coacervate) and the other phase exists as a highly dilute colloidal phase. The term "coacervate" essentially means "to assemble together or cluster" and the coacervate droplets typically have a diameter between 1 and 100 µm. A common example of this phenomenon is when aqueous solutions of the oppositely charged biopolymers gelatin and gum arabic are mixed; a gelatin–acacia coacervate has been used to encapsulate benzocaine in topical formulations.

Coacervates have been prepared between cationic tricyclic antidepressant (amitriptyline, imipramine, and doxepin) with anionic bile salts (sodium cholate, sodium deoxycholate) and sodium laurylsulphate (Stott et al., 1996). As with other ion-pair systems, drug partitioning into human skin membranes was improved by the coacervates, though flux enhancements were again modest.

3.4.3   Eutectic Systems/Depression of Permeant Melting Point

The General Solubility Equation is a quantitative structure property relationship-based model that uses the melting point and log P of a chemical substance to predict the aqueous solubility of non-ionisable chemical compounds (Ali et al., 2012). The equation has undergone various revisions – for example, Jain and Yalkowski (2001) – who related the intrinsic aqueous solubility of an un-ionised organic compound to its melting point (MP) and octanol–water partition coefficient as:

$$\text{Log solubility} = 0.5 - 0.01(\text{MP} - 25) - \log P_{\text{octanol–water}}$$

Which can be rearranged to give:

$$\text{Log}(\text{solubility} \times \text{partition coefficient}) = 0.55 - 0.01(\text{MP} - 25)$$

This approach was subsequently used to predict oral drug absorption (Chu and Yalkowski, 2009) and, in essence, shows that the lower the melting point of the drug, the greater the product of the solubility and partition coefficient – in general, low-melting compounds will be better absorbed than high-melting compounds.

It is well-known that pure enantiomers of chiral compounds usually possess different melting points to their racemic mixtures, and hence the lower melting forms can be selected to improve transdermal delivery. Thus, by selection of a lower melting form, enhanced delivery of chiral β-blockers was possible, and a similar approach was useful for improving delivery of chiral penetration enhancers to human stratum corneum (Mackay et al., 2001).

One method by which the melting point of a drug delivery system can be reduced is by eutectic formation. A binary eutectic is a mixture of two components that do not interact to form a new chemical compound, but which at a certain ratio inhibit the crystallisation process of one another. This results in a system that possesses a lower melting point than either of the two components, and the lowest melting point composition is described as the eutectic composition, as shown in Figure 3.9.

The first commercially successful eutectic formulation for topical use was EMLA cream, a eutectic mixture of the local anaesthetics lidocaine and prilocaine. As with other approaches such as prodrugs, combining the melting point depression effect with a chemical penetration enhancer has been explored. Thus, the melting point depression effect from eutectics generated using between ibuprofen and a series of terpene penetration enhancers was evaluated (Stott et al., 1998); most useful was a system

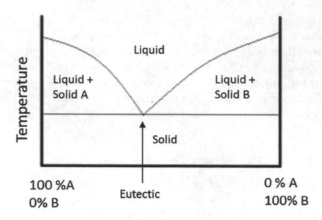

FIGURE 3.9 A phase diagram for a binary mixture of compounds A and B showing that they generate a low-melting eutectic mixture at a specific composition.

formed between the drug and the enhancer thymol, which generated a eutectic system that melted at 32°C (i.e., at around skin temperature). More complex behaviour was reported for propranolol with fatty acids where eutectic systems were formed between propranolol with an addition complex formed between propranolol and the enhancer capric acid (Stott et al., 2001). Terpenes have been used to form eutectic mixtures with other drugs, for example, lidocaine with thymol or menthol that provided compositions with melting points near or below skin temperature, and testosterone with menthol.

The mechanism for enhanced delivery from eutectic systems remains unclear. Naturally, the inclusion of an enhancer can modify the stratum corneum barrier properties as described previously. However, simply considering the melting point depression effect, at a gross level, it is clear that the lower melting point improves transdermal drug delivery, as predicted from the General Solubility Equation and shown experimentally for chiral compounds. In a eutectic mixture, the system has a lower melting point, but the permeant remains the original molecule of, for example, lidocaine. This parent molecule has the same properties as if in a simple saturated aqueous solution. Thus, the permeant melting point is not truly modified unless the permeant traverses the tissue with the counter molecule in the same proportion to the eutectic composition. Additionally, partitioning behaviour between the eutectic system and the skin probably affects permeation enhancement. However, by using a eutectic "liquid" saturated formulation, maximal thermodynamic activity in the donor phase can be maintained.

3.4.4 SUPERSATURATION

Chapter 2 described the mathematical principles underlying transdermal drug delivery and, in Section 2.5.2, considered the role of the thermodynamic activity of the permeant in the donor vehicle. Briefly, when delivered from a vehicle that does not itself affect the skin membrane, then Equation 2.10 gave:

$$J = \frac{DC_0}{h} \tag{2.10}$$

where J is the flux of the permeant, D is the diffusion coefficient of the permeant in the membrane, C_0 is the concentration of the permeant in the first layer of the membrane (at the skin surface, in contact with the donor solution), and h is the membrane thickness. This equation can be rewritten such that flux J (per unit area) can be described by:

$$J = \frac{D\alpha}{\gamma h} \tag{2.11}$$

where α is the thermodynamic activity of the drug in the vehicle, D is again the diffusion coefficient of the permeant, h remains the membrane thickness, and γ is the effective activity coefficient of the drug in the membrane. Analogous to the concentration term in Equation 2.10, Equation 2.11 shows that in order to obtain the maximum flux, the highest possible thermodynamic activity should be used. In essence, maximal flux is obtained when a saturated solution (thermodynamic activity of 1) is applied to the skin surface.

However, supersaturation can occur when the thermodynamic activity of the permeant in the vehicle exceeds 1, and so the concentration is essentially greater than the equilibrium solubility value. Many topical formulations are likely to generate supersaturated states when used clinically; formulations (creams, gels, etc.) applied to skin are typically rubbed in and chaotic processes occur as initial formulations collapse on use. For example, when a hydroalcoholic gel is rubbed onto skin, then the alcohol tends to volatilise (and permeate) rapidly, leaving a system enriched with water as the delivery vehicle. For a poorly water-soluble permeant, which has greater solubility in the alcohol, the loss of the "good" solvent from the formulation can elevate its thermodynamic activity in the residual formulation and so drive more drug into the skin.

Enhanced delivery using volatile solvents has long been recognised; as early as 1969, little penetration of fluocinolone acetonide and its acetate ester into human skin was reported when applied in non-volatile solvents, but with increasing incorporation of a volatile solvent, penetration increased up to 10-fold (Colman et al., 1969). The authors also noted that precipitation of the steroids prevented further increases in delivery. Supersaturated systems can also be generated by cooling a warm saturated solution back down to skin temperature, or by imbibing water from the skin into a formulation; the water can act as an antisolvent, and hence, the thermodynamic activity of the permeant in the changing vehicle increases.

Greater control over drug delivery can be generated from mixed solvent systems. As illustrated in Figure 3.10, ibuprofen is only slightly soluble in water, readily dissolves in ethanol, and solubility increases with increasing ethanol content in water:ethanol mixtures. If a water:ethanol system containing ibuprofen is diluted with water, then the solubility of the drug follows the dotted line in Figure 3.10. This forms a supersaturated state which is inherently thermodynamically unstable and so the supersaturated systems will crystallise and equilibrate to a saturated solution over time. However, the transient supersaturated system will provide greater drug flux compared to the saturated solution whilst the elevated thermodynamic activity is maintained.

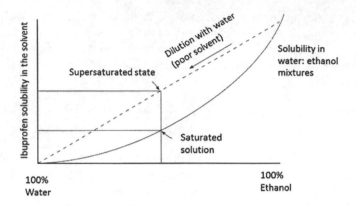

FIGURE 3.10 Illustration of the potential to generate supersaturated systems of ibuprofen from ethanol:water co-solvent systems.

As noted in the Colman et al. (1969) study and shown above, supersaturated states are inherently metastable and drive nucleation and crystal growth; the drug in excess of the solubility limit will, over time, crystallise out. Some supersaturated systems do, however, have prolonged stability, such as syrup (a supersaturated system of sugar). However, other systems can be stabilised by addition of appropriate excipients (antinucleating agents, typically polymers) for sufficient time to provide a clinically useful drug delivery system. Various anti-nucleating polymers, including hydroxypropylmethyl cellulose, polyvinylpyrrolidone, hydroxypropyl cellulose, and polyvinyl alcohol have been used in mixed solvent systems to stabilise supersaturated systems of oestradiol, piroxicam, fluocinonide, and ibuprofen which enhanced drug flux through human skin both *in vitro* and *in vivo*. As would be predicted from the theory, approximate linear relationships between the degree of supersaturation (or, more accurately, the increase in permeant thermodynamic activity) and the flux were reported, in other words, if the supersaturated state was at double the saturated solubility (2 degrees of saturation, thermodynamic activity = 2), then flux approximately doubles. Given that the supersaturated states are thermodynamically unstable, even with anti-nucleants, recrystallisation occurs over time. Further, thermodynamic instability increases with increasing degrees of supersaturation and so systems with degrees of supersaturation in excess of ~20 tend to be too unstable to use. Interestingly, as large molecular weight materials, the polymeric stabilisers are unable to enter the stratum corneum and so, with rapid ingress of the drugs into the tissue at levels in excess of the vehicle solubility, it appears that the stratum corneum components themselves are offering some inhibition of recrystallisation in the tissue (Megrab et al., 1995).

Given the instability of supersaturated systems formed from co-solvents, alternative formulations have been explored using the same principles. Water-free microemulsion bases saturated with bupranolol were applied to rabbit skin under occlusion; the occlusion led to water uptake into the base via transepidermal water loss through which the base converted into a microemulsion in which the drug was supersaturated as a result of decreasing solubility of the drug with increasing water content

(Kemken et al., 1992). More recently, a hydrophilic matrix containing ethanol was used to generate supersaturation of diclofenac (Benaouda et al., 2012). As ethanol evaporated, the matrix self-assembled and prevented drug recrystallisation from its supersaturated state for over 24 hours. Beclomethasone dipropionate was deposited onto human skin from a metered dose aerosol (MDA) containing the hydrofluoroalkane propellant 134a, ethanol and polyvinylpyrrolidone (Reid et al., 2009). With the steroid sub-saturated in the formulation, the time taken to generate a supersaturated state on the skin surface varied with ethanol content in the MDA. By increasing the volatile solvent content and drug concentration in the formulation, a supersaturated state could be formed on actuation, but the drug crystallised very rapidly on the skin surface, whereas with lower ethanol contents, achieving supersaturation on the skin surface took up to 30 minutes. A similar approach was used to enhance delivery of the corticosteroid betamethasone valerate into human skin; again using the hydrofluoroalkane propellant 134a with ethanol, polyvinylpyrrolidone, and polyethylene glycol, the spray deposited >6 times more drug into the skin compared to delivery from a commercial cream (Reid et al., 2013). The technology, known as MedSpray® incorporating terbinafine has also been shown to be clinically effective (Brown et al., 2013). A novel aerosol foam formulation has been described to deliver two active ingredients into skin (Lind et al., 2016). Calcipotriene and betamethasone dipropionate were fully dissolved in a dimethyl ether-containing aerosol foam formulation. After spraying, the ether rapidly evaporated, leading to the formation of supersaturated states with no evidence of crystals of either drug up to 26 h post-application. Both drugs had significantly greater *in vitro* skin penetration and increased bioavailability when compared to a conventional ointment.

REFERENCES

Ali, J., Camilleri, P., Brown, M.B., Hutt, A.J., and Kirton, S.B. (2012). Revisiting the general solubility equation: *in silico* prediction of aqueous solubility incorporating the effect of topographical polar surface area. *J. Chem. Inf. Model.* 52: 420–428.

Arezki, N.R., Williams, A.C., Cobb, A.J.A., and Brown, M.B. (2017). Design, synthesis and characterisation of linear unnatural amino acids for skin moisturisation. *Int. J. Cosmet. Sci.* 39: 72–82.

Aungst, B.J. (1989). Structure-effect studies of fatty acid isomers as skin penetration enhancers and skin irritants. *Pharm. Res.* 6: 244–247.

Aungst, B.J., Rogers, N.J., and Shefter, E. (1986). Enhancement of naloxone penetration through human skin in vitro using fatty acids, fatty alcohols, surfactants, sulfoxides and amides. *Int. J. Pharm.* 33: 225–234.

Barry, B.W. (1991). Lipid-protein-partitioning theory of skin penetration enhancement. *J. Control. Release* 15: 237–248.

Barry, B.W. (2004). Breaching the skin's barrier to drugs. *Nat. Biotechnol.* 22: 165–167.

Benaouda, F., Brown, M.B., Martin, G.P., and Jones, S.A. (2012). Triggered in situ drug supersaturation and hydrophilic matrix self-assembly. *Pharm. Res.* 29: 3434–3442.

Benaouda, F., Jones, S.A., Martin, G.P., and Brown, M.B. (2016). Localized epidermal drug delivery induced by supramolecular solvent structuring. *Pharm. Res.* 13: 65–72.

Björklund, S., Nowacka, A., Bouwstra, J.A., Sparr, E., and Topgaard, D. (2013). Characterization of stratum corneum molecular dynamics by natural-abundance ^{13}C solid-state NMR. *PLoS One.* DOI:10.1371/journal.pone.0061889

Blank, I.H. (1952). Factors which influence the water content of the stratum corneum. *J. Invest. Dermatol.* 18: 433–440.

Blank, I.H. (1953). Further observations on factors which influence the water content of the stratum corneum. *J. Invest. Dermatol.* 21: 259–269.

Brown, M.B., Evans, C.E., Muddle, A., Turner, R., Lim, S.T., and Traynor, M. (2013). Efficacy, tolerability and consumer acceptability of terbinafine topical spray versus terbinafine topical solution: a phase IIa, randomised, observer-blind, comparative study. *Am. J. Clin. Dermatol.* 14: 413–419.

Chu, K.A. and Yalkowski, S.H. (2009). An interesting relationship between drug absorption and melting point. *Int. J. Pharm.* 373: 24–40.

Colman, M.F., Poulsen, B.J., and Higuchi, T. (1969). Enhancement of percutaneous absorption by the use of volatile: non-volatile systems as vehicles. *J. Pharm. Sci.* 58: 1098–1102.

Dragicevic, N. and Maibach, H.I. (2015). *Percutaneous Penetration Enhancers, Chemical Methods in Penetration Enhancement; Modification of the Stratum Corneum*. Berlin: Springer–Verlag.

Feldman, R.J. and Maibach, H.I. (1965). Penetration of ^{14}C hydrocortisone through normal skin. *Arch. Dermatol.* 91: 661–666.

Hadgraft, J. and Lane, M.E. (2016). Drug crystallization – implications for topical and transdermal delivery. *Expert Opin. Drug Deliv.* 13: 817–830.

Hadgraft, J., Peck, J., Williams, D.G., Pugh, W.J., and Allan, G. (1996). Mechanisms of action of skin penetration enhancers / retarders: azone and analogues. *Int. J. Pharm.* 141: 17–25.

Horita, A. and Weber, L.J. (1964). Skin penetrating property of drugs dissolved in dimethyl sulphoxide (DMSO) and other vehicles. *Life Sci.* 3: 1389–1395.

Jacob, S.W., Bischel, M., and Herschler, R.J. (1964). Dimethyl sulphoxide: effects on the permeability of biologic membranes (preliminary report). *Curr. Ther. Res.* 6: 193–198.

Jain, N. and Yalkowsky, S.H. (2001). Estimation of the aqueous solubility I: application to organic nonelectrolytes. *J. Pharm. Sci.* 90: 234–252.

Karande, P., Jain, A., Arora, A., Ho, M.J., and Mitragotri, S. (2007). Synergistic effects of chemical enhancers on skin permeability: a case study of sodium lauroylsarcosinate and sorbitan monolaurate. *Eur. J. Pharm. Sci.* 31: 1–7.

Karande, P., Jain, A., and Mitragotri, S. (2004). Discovery of transdermal penetration enhancers by high-throughput screening. *Nat. Biotechnol.* 22: 192–197.

Kemken, J., Ziegler, A., and Muller, B.W. (1992). Influence of supersaturation on the pharmacodynamic effect of bupranol after dermal administration using microemulsions as vehicle. *Pharm. Res.* 9: 554–558.

Lind, M., Nielsen, K.T., Schefe, L.H., Norremark, K., Eriksson, A.H., Norsgaard, H., Pedersen, B.T., and Petersson, K. (2016). Supersaturation of calcipotriene and betamethasone dipropionate in a novel aerosol foam formulation for topical treatment of psoriasis provides enhanced bioavailability of the active ingredients. *Dermatol. Ther.* 6: 413–425.

Mackay, K.M.B., Williams, A.C., and Barry, B.W. (2001). Effect of melting point of chiral terpenes on human stratum corneum uptake. *Int. J. Pharm.* 228: 89–97.

Megrab, N.A., Williams, A.C., and Barry, B.W. (1995). Oestradiol permeation through human skin and silastic membrane: effects of propylene glycol and supersaturation. *J. Control. Release* 36: 277–294.

Reid, M.L., Benaouda, F., Khengar, R., Jones, S.A., and Brown, M.B. (2013). Topical corticosteroid delivery into human skin using hydrofluoroalkane metered dose aerosol sprays. *Int. J. Pharm.* 452: 157–165.

Reid, M.L., Jones, S.A., and Brown, M.B. (2009). Transient drug supersaturation kinetics of beclomethasone dipropionate in rapidly drying films. *Int. J. Pharm.* 371: 114–119.

Scheuplein, R.J. (1965). Mechanism of percutaneous absorption. I. Routes of penetration and the influence of solubility. *J. Invest. Dermatol.* 45: 334–346.

Scheuplein, R.J. (1977). Permeability of the skin. In: Lee, D.H.K., Falk, H.L., Murphy, S.D., and Geiger, S.R. (Eds.), *Handbook of Physiology, Section 9: Reactions to Environmental Agents*. Bethesda, MD: American Physiological Society, Chapter 19, pp. 229–323.

Stoughton, R.B. and Fritsch, W.C. (1964). Influence of dimethyl sulphoxide on human percutaneous absorption. *Arch. Dermatol.* 90: 512–517.

Stott, P.W., Williams, A.C., and Barry, B.W. (1996). Characterization of complex coacervates of some tricyclic antidepressants and evaluation of their potential for enhancing transdermal flux. *J. Control. Release* 41: 215–227.

Stott, P.W., Williams, A.C., and Barry, B.W. (1998). Transdermal delivery from eutectic systems: enhanced permeation of a model drug, ibuprofen. *J. Control. Release* 50: 297–308.

Stott, P.W., Williams, A.C., and Barry, B.W. (2001). Mechanistic study into the enhanced transdermal permeation of a model β-blocker, propranolol, by fatty acids; a melting point depression effect. *Int. J. Pharm.* 219: 161–176.

Williams, A.C. (2007). Pharmaceutical solvents as vehicles for topical dosage forms. In: Augustijns, P. and Brewster, M.E. (Eds.), *Solvent Systems and Their Selection in Pharmaceutics and Biopharmaceutics*. New York, NY: Springer & AAPS Press, Chapter 13, pp. 403–426.

Williams, A.C. and Barry, B.W. (1989). Urea analogues in propylene glycol as penetration enhancers in human skin. *Int. J. Pharm.* 56: 43–50.

Williams, A.C. and Barry, B.W. (1991a). The enhancement index concept applied to terpene penetration enhancers for human skin and model lipophilic (oestradiol) and hydrophilic (5-fluorouracil) drugs. *Int. J. Pharm.* 74: 157–168.

Williams, A.C. and Barry, B.W. (1991b). Terpenes and the lipid-protein-partitioning theory of skin penetration enhancers. *Pharm. Res.* 8: 17–24.

Williams, A.C., Shatri, S.R.S., and Barry, B.W. (1998). Transdermal permeation modulation by cyclodextrins: a mechanistic study. *Pharm. Dev. Tech.* 3: 283–296.

Zhai, H.B. and Maibach, H.I. (1996). Effect of barrier creams: human skin in vivo. *Contact Dermatitis* 35: 92–96.

Zhao, H., Liu, C., Quan, P., Wan, X., Shen, M., and Fang, L. (2017). Mechanism study on ion-pair complexes controlling skin permeability: effect of ion-pair dissociation in the viable epidermis on transdermal permeation of bisoprolol. *Int. J. Pharm.* 532: 29–36.

4 Physical and Technological Modulation of Topical and Transdermal Drug Delivery

4.1 INTRODUCTION

It is readily apparent that there are varied topical and transdermal formulations and devices that have been developed, all of which have their own distinct features. Chemical approaches to topical and transdermal permeation modulation have been described in Chapter 3. However, the distinction and boundaries between "chemical" and "physical/technological" approaches (also known as "active" approaches) to permeation modulation are somewhat arbitrary; for example, there is certainly a degree of technological expertise used when preparing liposomal drug carriers which obviously use chemicals. However, the intention in this chapter is to examine strategies that reportedly physically or mechanically perturb or circumvent the stratum corneum barrier, such as microneedles, laser ablation, electroporation, or physically enhanced flux, such as iontophoresis. Other strategies that are considered include ultrasound (or sonophoresis), thermophoresis, needleless injection (the use of high-velocity particles), and the use of vesicular carriers. Whilst not an exhaustive list of permeation modulation strategies, the chapter covers the majority of approaches that have been, or that are currently being, researched and are not covered elsewhere.

4.2 VESICLES

Encapsulation of drugs and cosmetics into vesicular systems has been popular for numerous delivery routes, and many topical preparations utilise this technology. Humectants such as glycerol and urea, sunscreens, and tanning agents have all been formulated in vesicular delivery systems, and some of the larger cosmetic companies have sought patent protection for incorporating enzymes within vesicles for topical application. In terms of drugs, intravenously infused anti-cancer drugs are found in commercial liposomal formulations with encapsulation reducing side effects and providing better drug targeting since the agents (amphotericin B, daunorubicin, doxorubicin) extravasate from the blood supply to the tumours. Cilag AG marketed the first topical liposomal drug formulation in Switzerland in 1988; Pevaryl Lipogel contains 1% econazole in a liposomal gel formulation; however, there have been few others since then. Although topical liposomal drug formulations have not been hugely successful in commercial terms, the literature contains numerous research papers on the use of liposomes to deliver many diverse therapeutic agents to, and across, various membranes. In addition, there is a plethora of vesicle types that range from "standard" liposomes, composed primarily of a phospholipid, to niosomes prepared from non-ionic surfactants to PEGylated liposomes which increase residence time of the vesicle in the systemic circulation (as with the commercial daunoXome preparation of daunorubicin). The discussion below concentrates on four of the more common vesicle types of current interest for drug and cosmetic delivery to, and through, the skin, namely "standard" phospholipid liposomes and the more specialised variants ethosomes, niosomes, and highly deformable (or elastic) transfersomes.

4.2.1 Liposomes

Liposomes can essentially be regarded as lipid vesicles that fully enclose an aqueous volume. The lipid molecules are usually phospholipid, with or without cholesterol, and the lipids may be arranged in one or more bilayers. The lipid composition affects the properties of the resulting liposome, so, for example, the addition of relatively small amounts of cholesterol tends to stabilise the membrane and hence the liposome would be somewhat more rigid than a non-cholesterol containing vesicle. Liposomes can trap hydrophilic molecules within their aqueous regions, or they can incorporate lipophilic molecules within the membrane. Liposomes can be classified in many ways: for example, depending on their method of preparation, or depending on their size or by their lamellarity (how many bilayers formed by the phospholipids).

Many methods of liposome preparation are available. Most commonly, a thin film of lipids is deposited onto the walls of a vessel – for example, by evaporation of a volatile solvent containing the required proportions of lipids – before the film is rehydrated with water, buffer, or an aqueous solution containing the material to be entrapped. If the film is rehydrated at temperatures above the phase transition temperature of the lipids, then multi-lamellar vesicles (termed MLVs) will form spontaneously. These large structures, typically 0.1 to 10 μm in diameter, have multiple lipid bilayers surrounding the aqueous core. The size and lamellarity of these MLVs are difficult to control, and hence these structures are generally processed further; sonication or extrusion through membrane filters will reduce lamellarity to form large uni-lamellar vesicles (LUVs, generally 1 to 5 μm in diameter) or small uni-lamellar vesicles (SUVs, usually 0.1 to 0.5 μm diameter). A further filtration or dialysis step is usually used after preparing encapsulated liposomal formulations, to remove any free drug from the system.

The majority of the papers reporting liposomal drug application to the skin conclude that the payload within the vesicles is localised in the outer skin layers, particularly in the stratum corneum, but also possibly in the viable epidermis. Further, the studies generally show that little of the drug enters the deeper skin tissue or passes to the systemic circulation, since lower systemic drug loadings are given by liposomal formulations compared with solution formulations.

Various possible mechanisms exist for the enhanced drug uptake into the stratum corneum from liposomes. Some liposomes may adsorb onto and fuse with the skin surface. This collapse of the formulation on the tissue could alter (increase) the driving force for permeation of the liberated molecules and hence facilitate penetration into the tissue. Clearly, the collapse of the formulation on the skin surface raises a second possibility, in that the lipid bilayers form a second barrier on top of the skin, hence reducing permeation of the hydrophilic molecules that were encapsulated within the aqueous core. Additionally, collapse of the liposomes on the skin surface could not account for the increased delivery of large macromolecular drugs whose physicochemical properties do not favour transdermal permeation. An alternative mechanism for liposome action is that the vesicles penetrate into the stratum corneum to some extent before they fuse with stratum corneum lipids and thus release their payload. This mechanism would allow the drug content within the tissue to increase, providing a reservoir of the therapeutic agent that could be a macromolecule. Such a scheme would also explain the observation that the most efficacious liposomes are often those formed from stratum corneum lipids; presumably such lipids would enter stratum corneum lipid domains more readily and would then fuse with endogenous lipids. Another proposed mechanism involves liposomal targeting of the pilosebaceous units of the follicular route. Researchers propose that liposome structure, composition, and size will determine which individual or combination of the above mechanisms will be responsible for the drug delivery process.

4.2.2   Non-Ionic Surfactant Vesicles (Niosomes)

Many of the preparation procedures and principles described above apply to niosomes which are essentially liposomes prepared primarily from non-ionic surfactants. As with conventional liposomes prepared from phospholipids, the properties of niosomes can be modified by incorporation of other excipients, such as cholesterol, into the membrane and they can possess one or more lipid bilayers encapsulating an aqueous core. A diverse range of materials have been used to form niosomes such as sucrose ester surfactants and polyoxyethylene alkyl ether surfactants; many non-ionic surfactants have relatively low toxicities, cause less damage to skin membranes than ionic surfactants and, in the case of sucrose esters, are readily biodegraded.

Early work on niosomes originated mainly from the cosmetic industry from which the formation of non-ionic surfactant vesicles was first reported in the 1970s, with many drug delivery studies reported since. As with phospholipid liposomes, alteration of transdermal drug delivery across the bulk of the stratum corneum from non-ionic surfactant vesicles may result from different mechanisms:

- A potential penetration-enhancing effect of the surfactants. Penetration-enhancing effects would be expected from direct disruption of stratum corneum membrane lipids, as described in Chapter 3 (Section 3.2.2.7).
- Vesicle penetration into the outer skin layers/fusion with the tissue surface. It is feasible that the vesicles enter the outer layers of the stratum corneum before fusing with lipid bilayers within the membrane.
- Vesicle collapse on the skin surface with two possible consequences; increasing the thermodynamic activity of the drug on the skin surface or forming an additional barrier layer on the tissue surface that could inhibit drug flux.

As before, the mechanism or combination of mechanisms described above that are responsible for any modulation will be governed by the physicochemical properties of the permeant, vehicle, and lipid used in the formulation.

Niosomes offer potential benefits over liposomes prepared from phospholipids. The components tend to be easier to source at a level and quality commensurate with that required for clinical manufacture, have less inherent toxicity, and would generally be less irritating to the skin. Both liposomes and niosomes are versatile in their compositions, sizes, and entrapment efficiencies, though to date, there is clearly a greater body of literature data behind phospholipid formulations compared to niosome systems.

4.2.3 Highly Deformable (or Elastic) Liposomes-Transfersomes®

As described previously, it is widely accepted that liposomes have a localising effect within the skin, forming a reservoir in the outer tissue layers whilst reducing permeation through the membrane and hence reducing systemic permeant loads. However, the possibility that intact vesicles can permeate through skin membranes to carry encapsulated material into the systemic circulation remains highly controversial. Nevertheless, over the last few decades, such a claim has been made for a new class of highly deformable (or elastic or ultraflexible) liposomes that have been termed Transfersomes. These vesicles comprise a phospholipid (e.g., phosphatidylcholine) as their main ingredient with 10 to 24 w/w% of a surfactant added. It is reported that the surfactant (e.g., sodium cholate or deoxycholate) has a high radius of curvature that acts as an "edge activator" and gives flexibility to the liposome. The formulation also typically contains 3 to 10% ethanol, and the final aqueous lipid suspension has a total lipid concentration of 4 to 10%.

Traditional liposomes, typically 200–400 nm in diameter, are too big to fit within the intercellular lipid domains of the stratum corneum. However, Transfersomes, as ultraflexible vesicles, are claimed by Cevc et al. (Cevc and Blume, 1992, 2001; Cevc, 1996, 2012; Cevc et al., 1996, 1997; Cevc and Vierl, 2010) to be able to squeeze through a pore that is only 1/10th of the vesicle diameter – in other words, through a pore around 20 nm in diameter. The driving force for the vesicles entering the skin is proposed to be xerophobia – the tendency to avoid dry surroundings. A hydration gradient exists across human skin *in vivo*, from around 20% at the outer surface (depending on environmental conditions) to approaching 100% within the skin at the epidermal–dermal junction. The principal component of the highly deformable vesicle is a phospholipid which requires hydration to remain in its most stable maximally swollen state. It is claimed that if a finite dose of Transfersomes is placed on the skin surface, the formulation will dry and the vesicles will start to partially dehydrate. The surfactant in the formulation (the edge activator) then accumulates at the high stress sites within the vesicles and so forms a highly curved area of the vesicle which, to maintain stability, will then move through the narrow skin pores to the more hydrated environment within the deeper skin strata. Traditional liposomes are unable to deform and hence cannot penetrate the tissue; they are thus confined to the outer layers of the stratum corneum, or fuse with the skin surface as they dry.

Many of the consequent properties for Transfersome formulations thus derive from this proposed mechanism of action. For example, the formulation can only work if applied as a finite dose under non-occluded conditions; the formulation must be allowed to dry out to cause the vesicles to enter the skin, and there must be a hydration gradient across the membrane to generate the driving force whereby occluded conditions fully hydrate the stratum corneum. For similar reasons, *in vitro* experiments that tend to use a fully hydrated membrane will not be appropriate for examining drug delivery from highly deformable vesicles.

The literature reports concerning the efficacy of these highly deformable liposomes generated much interest and controversy, as many of the claims contradict established knowledge for traditional liposomal systems. The inventors claimed that the vesicles penetrated into the deeper skin strata intact, and even into the systemic circulation.

4.2.4 ETHOSOMES

Ethosomes are comprised of phospholipids, as with traditional liposomal formulations, but also incorporate high levels of an alcohol, usually ethanol, and water. The use of ethanol, typically at 30% in the formulation, creates a "soft" vesicle that can be modified in terms of size and lamellarity, as above. They have also been shown to be capable of delivering compounds to the deeper skin layers or to the systemic circulation, and they can be designed to improve transdermal delivery of lipophilic or hydrophilic molecules.

The mechanisms of action of these carriers are not clear. Clearly, the formulations contain high levels of ethanol, which has previously been shown to be a penetration enhancer (see Chapter 3, Section 3.2.2.6), as well as phospholipids which also have the potential to disrupt the intercellular lipid domains to facilitate permeation. However, controls such as a hydroethanolic solution of the permeant appear less effective for promoting drug delivery than the ethosomes, suggesting that the vesicular structure and permeant entrapment is important for efficacy. The vesicular bilayers are flexible and have a low melting transition, and it is feasible that this flexibility is again essential for the deep deposition into the stratum corneum lipid bilayers which may then be disrupted by the ethanol and phospholipid formulation components. The presence of high ethanol contents may suggest that the formulations pose a toxicity risk.

4.2.5 APPLICABILITY

Despite the advantages that have been described above, there are very few topical therapeutic liposomal preparations on the market. The sourcing of the required high purity and quality of lipids can be difficult and costly, whilst preparation and processing of vesicle-containing formulations, and especially those using more specialised lipids, is complex and requires even more specialised equipment when compared to, for example, creams and ointments – again with cost implications. Also, difficulties remain with loading drug into vesicles, and entrapment efficiencies can be low. Furthermore, physical stability issues with leakage of entrapped material and degradation of the vesicular structure can limit the use of liposomal preparations.

4.3 NANOSYSTEMS

Nanosystems or nanoparticles were first proposed in the late 1960s for use in drug delivery across the skin in the form of vaccinations. However, it wasn't until the mid-1990s that they gained sufficient attention to require the *Encyclopaedia of Pharmaceutical Technology* to define them as "solid colloidal particles ranging in size from 1–1000 nm, consisting of macromolecular materials that can be used as drug carriers in/to which the active is either dissolved, entrapped or encapsulated or sorbed". The first commercially available nanoparticle product appeared in the US and was an injectable suspension of human serum albumin nanoparticles containing paclitaxel. Although the application of nanosystems or nanoparticles for drug to delivery to and across the skin has been relatively slow, there is now a plethora of literature available on the subject, with quantum dots, metal and metal oxide nanoparticles, dendrimers, carbon nanotubes, nanoemulsions, lipid-based colloidal nanosystems, and flexible nanovesicles all attracting attention.

The mechanisms by which such nanoparticles achieve drug permeation across and to the skin still remain a subject of intense debate. Nevertheless, the properties of nanoparticles that could explain enhanced drug delivery across the stratum corneum or follicular uptake include their size, shape, charge, surface properties, and aggregation state. In addition, the vehicle in which they are formulated and the disease state of the skin to which they are applied could also both play a role.

Lipid nanoparticles (LNs) are the nanoparticle systems currently receiving the greatest attention. LNs are colloidal dispersions composed of a dispersed lipid phase stabilised by an emulsifier/emulsifier system, with a size of between 10 nm and 10 um. If solid lipids are utilised, then the LNs are specified as solid lipid nanoparticles (SLNs), and if a mixture of liquid lipids is incorporated, then nanolipid carriers (NLCs) result. Both of these colloidal systems may increase the solubility or bioavailability of a drug, protect a drug from degradation caused by light or oxygen, and also provide a means of achieving enhanced drug delivery. Nonetheless, as NLCs have a fluid phase incorporated into the nanoparticle, the lipids' spatial structure allows greater drug loading and drug protection compared to SLNs. NLCs and SLNs are reported to have a similar mechanism of drug permeation enhancement, with occlusion and mixing between the formulation and skin lipids being largely responsible. However, the presence of the liquid lipid component in NLCs provides increased solubilisation, and consequent increased drug release and loading into the stratum corneum, resulting in greater delivery compared to SLNs. Both systems have the benefit of being manufactured under scalable processes such as high-pressure homogenisation, microemulsion technologies, and ultrasonication, along with their biocompatibility and non-toxicity because they can be prepared from Generally Recognised as Safe (GRAS) or Inactive Ingredients Database (IID) excipients. However, although both systems have been proposed as platforms for potential reformulation of known drugs to extend product lifecycle, the costs of the ingredients and manufacture when compared to more conventional dosage forms cannot be ignored.

4.4 NEEDLELESS INJECTION

The concept of a needleless injection is not new – indeed the U.S. military experimented with such devices for vaccination during the Vietnam War – but it is only since the early 1990s, when Professor Bellhouse, Head of the University of Oxford's Medical Engineering Unit, developed a gas powered "gun" to fire particles into skin, that many alternative devices and formulations have been proposed to deliver varied agents to and through the tissue based on both liquid (Ped-O-Jet®, Iject® Biojector2000®, Medi-jector®, Tjet®, and Intraject®) and powder systems (PMED™ device, formerly known as the Powderject® injector). Transdermal delivery is achieved by firing the liquid or solid (drug powder alone or engineered particles, including gold) at supersonic speeds (100 to 200 m/s) through the outer layers of the skin using a suitable energy source, such as a helium gas cylinder. Amongst the many potential benefits claimed of this technology are:

- Pain-free administration can be achieved, since particles fired into the skin are too small to trigger pain receptors within the tissue – though some sensation may be felt.
- Specific skin strata can be targeted. This is beneficial during, for example, vaccination when delivery to the viable epidermal cells is desired.
- The fear of needles is avoided.
- Accurate dosing can be achieved.
- The technology should reduce accidental needle-stick injuries and should avoid infection or splash-back from bodily fluids.

However, there are still some issues to be resolved when delivering materials to the body via this technology, including:

- Dosage accuracy may be lower than from a needle. Though a perceived advantage above, clearly delivery of a fixed volume via a needle to a specific tissue (e.g., the muscle) may be more accurate than firing particles through the skin to the tissue.
- Careful use of the device (compliance) may be necessary to avoid particles "bouncing off" the skin surface and if the device is not held vertically then the dose may escape or could penetrate the skin to differing degrees.
- The thickness of stratum corneum and other skin layers varies between individuals and hence penetration depth of particles could vary.
- The external environment could affect delivery. For example, delivery through hydrated skin could differ to that through less hydrated skin.
- Particle delivery through the stratum corneum has been described as akin to throwing rocks through a brick wall. Regulatory bodies need be assured that there is no lasting damage to the stratum corneum structure and that there is no significant risk of bacterial infection through the "holes" left in the stratum corneum. In defence of the system, it is readily apparent that the "holes" would be smaller than those left by a needle.

Nevertheless, the types of drug or biologic that have been investigated for delivery by such systems are wide and varied and include lidocaine, antibiotics, calcitonin, inulin, insulin, interferon, somatropin, hGH, and DNA vaccines (influenza A, hepatitis B). However, despite over 15 years of research, the commercial success of such systems is distinctly lacking.

4.5 PHYSICAL AVOIDANCE OF THE STRATUM CORNEUM

As the major barrier to transdermal and topical drug delivery of most agents resides in the stratum corneum, efforts have been directed at circumventing this layer by "physical means", and include the use of microneedles and ablation.

4.5.1 LASER ABLATION

Removal of the stratum corneum has long been known to increase the flux of drugs permeating through skin, and many methods have been used to remove this outer layer from the underlying tissue, such as tape stripping or the use of cyanoacrylate adhesives. A more controlled method to remove the stratum corneum is via the use of lasers. As the use of lasers in medicine in general and within dermatology in particular has increased, so has laser precision and accuracy. Various lasers (excimer, erbium:yttrium scandium gallium garnet, erbium:yttrium aluminium garnet) have been used to ablate the stratum corneum and facilitate the delivery of both lipophilic and hydrophilic drugs, and by confining ablation to this outer layer, the tissue will regenerate from below. The technique allows highly specific targeting for local therapy, but removal of large areas of tissue to permit systemic delivery is more questionable. Commercially, a hand-held portable laser device was developed by Norwood Abbey Ltd. (Victoria, Australia) to reduce the time to onset of action of lidocaine and was approved by the U.S. and Australian regulatory bodies. However, the device did not gain any significant market traction.

4.5.2 OTHER ABLATION METHODS

Other techniques for the selective removal of outer skin layers have been used for improving drug delivery – for example, chemical peels can remove layers varying from the superficial stratum corneum to the epidermis, or even to the dermal tissue. Radiofrequency (RF) thermal ablation involves placing a thin, needle-like electrode directly into the skin and applying high frequency alternating current (~100 kHz) which produces microscopic pathways in the stratum corneum through which drugs can permeate. Adhesive tape can be used to sequentially remove stratum corneum layers. Additionally, dermabrasion can be used to remove the stratum corneum, or even the deeper skin layers; it is akin to simply using "sandpaper" on the skin, by firing aluminium oxide crystals at localised areas of the skin to remove tissue. As with the laser treatment, flux of both lipophilic and hydrophilic molecules would be expected to increase, but at present the technology appears only suited to local (i.e., in the vicinity of the application, not systemic) drug delivery. One apparently successful approach has to be the use of microporation with a dry patch. In Nitto's PassPort® Active Transdermal Platform, a disposable portable device ablates the skin to create micropores in the stratum corneum through which small APIs and biologic drugs can penetrate down into the systemic circulation.

4.5.3 MICRONEEDLES

Microneedles can puncture the skin to create micron-sized channels and can be used to facilitate both topical and transdermal delivery of molecules with diverse physicochemical properties (small molecular weight drugs to biologics) across the skin.

Microneedle systems are comprised of multiple microscopic projections typically assembled on one side of a supporting base or patch, generally ranging from 25 to 2000 µm in height, 50 to 250 µm in base width, and 1 to 25 µm in tip diameter. The needles are designed to be of a suitable length, width, and shape to avoid nerve contact when inserted into skin layers. They are usually designed in arrays to create transient aqueous conduits across the skin, thereby enhancing flux of the molecules ranging from small hydrophilic drugs to macromolecules, including low molecular weight heparins, insulin, and vaccines in a pain-free manner. Besides the aspect of pain-free delivery, there are many other advantages of microneedle technologies which include:

- They should not cause bleeding.
- They reduce the topical and transdermal dosing variability.
- They have potential for self-administration.
- They have the potential to overcome and reduce instances of accidental needle-stick injuries and the risk of transmitting infections.

Generally, there are four types of microneedle systems used in drug delivery to and across the skin. These are solid, coated, dissolvable, and hollow systems, illustrated in Figure 4.1.

Hollow microneedles are used to deliver drug solutions via the "poke and flow" method where the microneedle is inserted and then a solution is transported (actively

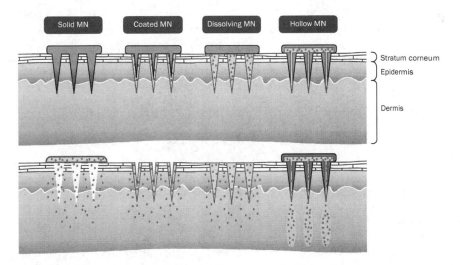

FIGURE 4.1   **(See color insert.)** Illustration of the principal types of microneedles available and their typical dosing sites.

or passively) through it in much the same way as a hypodermic syringe. For the "poke and patch" type microneedle systems, a solid microneedle system is used to create microchannels or holes in the skin. The microneedle array is then removed and a formulation (e.g., patch or semi-solid) is then applied over the site of the pores. Microneedles can also be coated with the drug that requires delivery, known as the "coat and poke" system, and results in a one-step process allowing for rapid drug delivery. For the "poke and release" system, the microneedles are fabricated from biocompatible materials (e.g., poly-L-lactic acid, poly-glycolic acid, poly-carbonate, poly-lactic-co-glycolic acid [PLGA], polydimethylsiloxane, a copolymer of methyl vinyl ether and maleic anhydride, carboxymethylcellulose, maltose, dextrin, and galactose) and the drug itself. When applied, they detach, and dissolution in the case of dissolvable microneedles or swelling in the case of hydrogel microneedles occurs, allowing drug release. This strategy eliminates the need for sharps disposal and the possibility of accidental reuse of the system.

As would be expected with such systems, flux enhancement is dramatic and several companies have been working towards the development of microneedle-based drug or vaccine products, including 3M, Clearside Biomedical, NanoPass Technologies, Corium International, TheraJect, Circassia, Radius Health, Lohmann Therapeutic Systems (LTS), and Zosano Pharma, with the first three commercially marketed microneedle-based products being Intanzia® for influenza vaccine (Sanofi), Micronjet® for intradermal delivery of liquid vaccines and drugs (Nanopass), and the 3M Microneedle Drug Delivery Systems, which includes Hollow Microneedle and Solid Microneedle technology for the delivery of vaccines and difficult to deliver biologics.

Nevertheless, despite microneedles being a promising strategy for enhancing drug transport across skin, there are some reported limitations such as: (i) unlikely to be useful in diseased skin, (ii) the small size of the needles limits the therapeutic delivery rates of high-dose and low-potency molecules, (iii) it is very important to consider the variations of skin thickness while designing microneedles, since this could affect the natural behaviour of the barrier and hence influence the drug delivery, (iv) microneedle tips can be broken off and left under the skin, (v) microneedles can be difficult to apply on the skin, and (vi) product sterility and scale-up manufacture to industrial levels is complex. In addition, as a new technology, limited data are available concerning transient and long-term skin damage (e.g., erythema, oedema, immune response), or on the potential for microbial contamination – though with such small needles, it may be expected that there is a reduced risk of infection as compared with a standard needle.

4.6   ULTRASOUND

Ultrasound is an oscillating sound pressure wave that has long been used for many research areas, including physics, chemistry, biology, engineering, and others, in a wide range of frequencies. For skin delivery, ultrasound, sonophoresis, or phonophoresis can be defined as the transport of drugs across the skin by application of ultrasound perturbation at frequencies of 20 kHz to 16 MHz which have sufficient intensity to reduce the resistance of skin. The drug may be delivered simultaneously while ultrasound is being applied, or the skin may be pre-treated with ultrasound followed by application of the drug.

The use of ultrasound has resulted in the effective delivery of various categories and classes of drugs (including hydrophilic and large molecular weight drugs) regardless of their electrical characteristics. However, the mechanism of action is still not fully defined. Ultrasonic energy can have various effects on biological tissues, the scale of which again varies upon factors such as ultrasound frequency and intensity. High-intensity ultrasound can warm up the tissue when used to deliver permeants across the skin, although whether the temperature increase at the skin surface is sufficient to impact drug flux requires further research. Low-frequency ultrasound, as used in phonophoresis can cause cavitation (the collapse of gas bubbles in liquid media as the ultrasound pressure waves pass through at the coupling medium/stratum corneum boundary) that could disturb the intercellular lipid bilayers. The cavitational effects vary inversely with ultrasound frequency and directly with ultrasound intensity. At frequencies greater than 1 MHz, the density variations occur so rapidly that a small gaseous nucleus cannot grow, and cavitational effects cease. As such, when using ultrasound for therapeutic means, it is essential to control and optimise numerous variables, including the ultrasound intensity, pulse length, and frequency, and it is also necessary to use the correct contact medium (such as a gel) to efficiently transfer the ultrasound energy to the body, since air reflects ultrasound. In addition, although the mechanism of action dictates that the stratum corneum is "damaged" through the creation of pores or pits in its surface, it is believed that its barrier properties return to normal within 24 h.

Many of the early studies focused on locally acting agents, such as delivery of steroids for arthritis, anti-inflammatory agents, and local anaesthetics, whilst later, macromolecules including insulin (molecular weight around 6000 Da), gamma interferon (~17,000 Da), and erythropoeitin (~48,000 Da) were all investigated with some success. The first commercially available transdermal ultrasound device, SonoPrep® (Sontra Medical) was approved in 2004 by the FDA for the delivery of local dermal anaesthesia, but had limited/no success. Although research in the area still continues, commercially there has been little development over the last 15 years, which may be explained by the lack of success of SonoPrep®, but perhaps also the reported unwanted effects such as minor tingling, irritation, and burning of skin (although these can often be reduced or eliminated by optimising important parameters such as frequency, intensity, pulse length, and application time).

4.7   ELECTRICAL METHODS

Several of the permeation modulation strategies described above could be incorporated under the general banner of "electrical methods". Some of the methodologies described below electrically drive molecules through the skin (such as iontophoresis) whereas others use electrical means for creating pores within the membrane (e.g., electroporation). Many review articles and book chapters deal specifically with some of these techniques. It is the intention here to give a broad overview of the scope of enhancement and the utility of these techniques for various classes of therapeutic agents.

4.7.1 IONTOPHORESIS

Iontophoresis uses an electrical potential gradient to facilitate drug delivery into the skin. Though a well-established technique that was used in the 19th century, iontophoresis has yet to be widely adopted, although it has found some clinical application. Iontophoresis uses an electrical supply terminating with an anode (positive electrode) and a cathode (negative electrode). The (usually charged) drug is dissolved in a suitable vehicle and is placed in contact with the electrode of the same polarity, with the second (grounding) electrode being placed elsewhere to complete the circuit. When the current flows, the drug is repelled from the electrode of similar polarity and is attracted towards the oppositely charge electrode, thus driving the drug into the skin.

Two primary mechanisms of action exist for increased drug delivery during iontophoresis. Electro-repulsion, as described above, where drug molecules are repelled by an electrode of similar polarity, is the principal mechanism operating. However, delivery of neutral molecules can also be enhanced through electro-osmosis. As the electric current is applied, endogenous ions within the skin also travel to the oppositely charged electrode. Sodium ions (Na^+) migrate to the cathode (negatively charged), and as they do so, they carry water with them. This net flow of water is related to the applied current, but is estimated at microlitres per hour, and can carry neutral molecules from the anode to the cathode. One further possibility is that the skin lipids may be damaged or disrupted to some degree by the applied current; most studies using human skin and "acceptable" current densities up to $0.5 \ mA/cm^2$ show no evidence for skin damage, but the literature contains reports where extravagant current densities are applied to the more fragile rodent membranes whereupon enhanced flux could be attributed to skin damage.

Iontophoretic conditions require optimisation for drug delivery on an individual basis. A prime concern is the selection of electrodes. Clearly the electrodes need to be prepared from conductive material, and inert materials such as platinum and stainless steel have been used. However, during iontophoresis, these inert electrodes generate H+ and OH- ions from water (electrolysis) that modifies the pH at the electrodes and the effects can be dramatic, which could result in skin irritation and/or drug degradation. It is now widely accepted that reversible electrodes are more suited for iontophoresis. These systems, such as silver/silver chloride electrodes, are essentially a metal in contact with a solution of its own ions which avoid electrolysis of water and hence the pH within the systems does not change.

The current density applied to the skin also affects delivery efficiency. It has been shown by many workers using diverse membranes for a variety of drugs that a linear relationship exists between the steady-state flux of a drug and the applied current. This linear relationship derives from the Nernst–Planck equation, although no account is taken of drug transport via electro-osmosis and hence some deviations from linearity between current density and flux may be expected. Generally, the current is limited to below 1 mA (commonly $0.5 \ mA/cm^2$) in order to facilitate patient comfort and consider safety concerns, as with increasing current, the risk of non-specific vascular reactions (vasodilatation) also increases. A direct current (DC) is generally used, since the switching of an alternating current (AC) will sequentially deliver and extract drug from the tissue. However, continuously applied direct current can, over time, polarise the skin, which then reduces the efficiency of delivery, and beyond 3 mins can cause local skin irritation or burns. To overcome these issues, a pulsed DC current can be applied so that the skin can depolarise and approach its normal electrical condition during the "off" phase between current pulses.

The nature of the vehicle from which the drug is being delivered must also be carefully controlled. As outlined above, many electro-processes can occur during iontophoresis and hence care must be taken with, for example, buffer selection. Buffers are often added to control the pH of the donor solution and are salt solutions containing small ions. As these ions are small, they are usually more mobile than the drug ions, especially if delivering peptides or proteins, and are more easily transported into the skin. This competition reduces flux of the therapeutic agent, and hence it is preferable to avoid the use of buffers in iontophoretic donor solutions, or to use buffer solutions containing large ions, such as HEPES buffer. The addition of buffer ions also increases the ionic strength of the donor solution, and it has been shown that an inverse relationship exists between ionic strength and drug delivery by iontophoresis. Control over donor solution pH is essential when delivering weak acids and weak bases in order to ensure that the molecules are present in their ionised form. Indeed, the proportion of ionised to un-ionised species can be selected by buffer pH with concomitant increases or decreases in drug flux.

As well as the electrical and formulation considerations for optimising iontophoretic delivery, permeant properties can also affect drug flux. Whilst polar neutral molecules can be delivered via electro-osmosis, and some component of this mechanism contributes to the flux of ionic molecules, electro-repulsion depends on the permeant charge. More accurately, charge density on the permeant is important. It may be expected that the higher charge density would give greater electro-repulsion and hence increase flux, or contrarily that the greater charge density on the cations gave stronger binding to negatively charged binding sites known to exist within the tissue, hence reducing flux. The influence of charge on iontophoretic transport is further complicated by modification of the skin barrier due to potential cation binding and also because of electro-osmotic water flow. As with conventional topical and transdermal drug delivery, a permeant's lipophilicity and molecular size can also be a governing factor in iontophoretic delivery, with research suggesting that for macromolecules above 12k Da, iontophoresis has limited applicability. The pKa of the material for delivery will also affect flux via pH and hence ionisation variations.

The uses of iontophoresis can be classified into therapeutic and diagnostic applications. The major advantage of iontophoresis in the latter is that there is no mechanical penetration or disruption of the skin involved in this approach, and it has been used in diagnosing cystic fibrosis and for monitoring blood glucose levels. Commercialised into a system that came to market, the GlucoWatch® extracts (reverse iontophoresis) and then quantifies glucose using an amperometric biosensor over 12 h with a 20 min lag time. A disadvantage with the system was that it required a once-daily calibration using the standard pinprick method, and this, along with the evolution of more responsive sensors often combined with insulin pumps, meant that the device very quickly lost its value. Iontophoresis alone is approved for treatment of hyperhidrosis (a condition characterised by excessive sweating) where tap water iontophoresis can provide symptomatic relief. With regard to drug delivery, Phoresor®, Lidosite®, E-trans®, Ionsys, and Zecuity are examples of commercially developed iontophoretic delivery systems, although it is probably fair to say that none to date have gained the market share that was hoped.

Nevertheless, in terms of therapy, iontophoresis is highly controllable, and can be switched off and on to give a rapid onset of action; iontophoresis lag times tend to be in the order of minutes, rather than the hours seen for passive transdermal drug delivery. Since delivery is related to the applied current, some of the biological variability inherent for passive strategies is reduced and so there is better inter- and intra-patient reproducibility of delivery. However, one major advantage is the ability to tailor delivery to the individual patients needs by simple manipulation of the dose (via the current density) and duration of delivery. Future developments are likely to see attempts to incorporate biofeedback mechanisms into iontophoretic devices to control and individualise dosage regimens.

4.7.2 Electroporation

Electroporation (or electropermeabilisation) is a long-established technique for permeabilising biological membranes and is widely used to introduce, for example, genetic material into bacterial cells. Typically, relatively high voltages (10 to 1000 V) are applied as pulses to the membranes for very short periods of time (typically micro- to milli-seconds). The pulses create transient aqueous pores in lipid membranes that permit DNA to be introduced into bacterial cells. In the electroporation of skin, the tissue is temporarily exposed to high intensities of electric pulses that lead to the formation of aqueous pores in the lipid bilayers of the stratum corneum, thus providing a direct pathway for drug absorption. Drug transport through these pores can be facilitated by three mechanisms: iontophoresis during the pulse, electro-osmosis, or by simple diffusion through the aqueous pores that remain open for some time after pulsing. Interestingly, the efficiency of electroporation in human skin is approximately 100 times less that in a microbial membrane; human stratum corneum has around 100 lipid bilayers for a molecule to traverse before reaching the epidermis.

As with other electrical methods, numerous operating parameters affect drug delivery. Electric pulses can be applied to the skin in various forms – exponentially decaying pulses or square wave pulses are common. Similarly, the applied voltage can be modified, as can the number and duration of the electric pulses; generally, increasing pulse conditions (length, intensity, number) increases permeability, although a threshold value is reached beyond which enhancement plateaus. In addition, electrode type can influence efficiency.

Usage of high voltage pulses (50–500 V) for short times of only one second have been shown to increase transport across the skin for different molecular weight drugs ranging from small to macromolecules of up to 40k Da. However, the main drawbacks are the lack of quantitative delivery, cell death with high fields, the questionable reversibility of the process, and potential damage to labile biologics.

4.8 HEAT (THERMOPHORESIS)

The use of heat as a strategy to enhance percutaneous absorption was reported in the 1960s and is generally known as thermophoresis. As mentioned previously, heat can be used in the form of thermal ablation (thermoporation, radio frequency, and lasers) for a short period at a very high temperature ($\geq 100°C$), until the tissues are vaporised and removal of the stratum corneum occurs prior to drug application. An alternative approach involves the use of chemical mixtures to produce heat which are concomitantly applied with the drug. This mode of delivery is non-invasive and involves the use of heat typically generated by chemical reaction ($<50°C$) applied locally for short duration to temporarily and reversibly disrupt the barrier properties of the stratum corneum, resulting in enhanced drug transport across skin. This approach is especially enticing when synergistically combined with chemical penetration enhancers so as to expand the range of drugs with diverse properties that can be delivered across the skin.

The number of marketed products utilising chemically generated heat to facilitate drug transport across the skin is very limited. Synera™/Rapydan™, a topical patch that combines lidocaine and tetracaine, using proprietary Controlled Heat-Assisted Drug Delivery (CHADD™) was licenced in the United States and Europe. The CHADD heating patch uses iron oxidation as a source of heat energy and is able to generate a skin surface temperature of 42°C for up to four hours, or even longer. It consists of an outer semi-permeable membrane that controls the temperature by allowing the ingress of oxygen to initiate iron oxidation. Below this outer semi-permeable membrane is a semi-synthetic air permeable pouch that contains heat-generating material: iron, carbon, sodium chloride, vermiculite, and water. The next layer is a pressure-sensitive skin adhesive layer. This is followed by a heat-sealable barrier film, which separates the formulation from the temperature control components. Other non-drug-containing and heat-generating patches on the market that utilise similar heat-generating material as CHADD include: Cura-Heat® Patches, Deep Heat Pain Relief Heat Patch, Nurofen® Express Heat Patches, ThermaCare®, and Voltarol® Thermal Patch Heat Patch. These patches are not used to deliver active drug molecules across skin but are rather used for their therapeutic heat to help reduce muscular and joint pains.

Bioré® Warming Anti-Blackhead cleanser, a topical cream which contains salicylic acid for the treatment of acne is available across Australia, Europe, and the United States. It consists of an anhydrous composition (e.g., surfactant, polymer, glycols, and zeolite) that generates heat in the presence of water. Within this product, heat is generated using zeolites, which are reportedly capable of heating the skin up to 47°C for less than one minute. More recently, supercooled salt solutions containing sodium acetate trihydrate and sodium thiosulfate pentahydrate have been identified as suitable phase-change materials with excellent ability to store heat, have high thermal conductivity, are relatively cheap, possess the ability to remain stable in the supercooled state for years, and are GRAS listed. Producing supercooled solutions involves: dissolving the phase-change material in a vehicle (such as water) with simultaneous heating, followed by cooling of the mixture to generate a supersaturated salt system that remains in solution. The latent heat stored within the system can be released by a liquid to solid phase change (recrystallisation), which can be initiated by introducing a nucleating agent. Like iron oxidation patches, supercooled systems are also commercially available as heat packs for various uses including muscle and joint pains, for example, ThermaClick Heat Pads.

Important parameters such as intensity and duration of heat (controlled by, for example, the mass/volume of heat-generating material and the presence of a trigger such as oxygen/nucleating agent) and exposure time are known to influence heat-facilitated percutaneous absorption. Other factors such the rate of crystallisation and the level of saturation are thought to be important parameters for phase-change materials. Therefore, these parameters can be manipulated and optimised for either local or systemic drug delivery, whilst avoiding cutaneous damage or patient discomfort. Whilst there are no regulatory limits on the intensity and duration of heat produced by thermophoretic delivery systems, the scarce information on temperatures tolerated by the skin would suggest that an appropriate range for thermophoretic delivery system would be 44–47°C. Consequently, most studies investigating heat-facilitated percutaneous absorption have employed temperatures of ≤45°C, which is within the physiologically tolerable range.

The mechanism by which heat enhances percutaneous drug delivery is not fully elucidated. However, heat may enhance percutaneous absorption by influencing the following parameters; the release of permeant from the formulation/vehicle, partitioning of the permeant into the stratum corneum and diffusion through it, and finally, partitioning from the stratum corneum to the viable epidermis and lower layers from where a permeant can be taken up systemically. Additionally, heat may reversibly disrupt the stratum corneum barrier at temperatures of ≤45°C by changing stratum corneum lipid organisation from an ordered state (orthorhombic) to a more disordered state (hexagonal), resulting in enhanced percutaneous delivery. Finally, raising the skin temperature is likely to increase cutaneous blood circulation, which leads to increased drug clearance into system circulation. This increase in drug clearance is likely to maintain a high concentration gradient from the formulation to the sink conditions in the dermis, which drives transdermal drug delivery.

Nevertheless, concerns have been raised about the suitability of heat-facilitated drug delivery due to the expense and size of the required packaging and the risk of dose variability and thermal burns, which could occur due to changes in air oxygen, humidity, and pressure; combined, these issues may explain their relative lack of commercial success.

4.9   COMBINED ENHANCEMENT STRATEGIES

The strategies described in Chapter 3 to modulate (usually enhance, occasionally retard) permeation though skin possess varying ranges of activity. Additionally, the approaches are at differing levels of maturity and hence whilst some are used commercially, others are more preliminary. For example, penetration enhancers such as ethanol are found in patches and other transdermal or topical formulations, but it is highly unlikely that a chemical penetration enhancer will ever be effective for the delivery of peptides, proteins, or DNA across the skin. Similarly, commercial attempts at iontophoretic delivery of peptides are yet to overcome the obstacles of skin irritation and drug damage. In order to improve the scale and utility of the strategies outlined above, several workers have combined the above approaches, primarily to deliver these large biological molecules. For example, a number of physical approaches such as sonophoresis, electroporation, ultrasound, and iontophoresis have been combined with microneedles in order to enhance permeation of drugs. In addition, combining active-transport strategies with chemical penetration enhancers is also popular. The potential benefits of modifying the bilayer lipid packing and/or the solvent nature of the skin to promote partitioning of the drug into the membrane, together with either electrically driving molecules across the tissue or further perturbing the skin lipids is attractive – exploiting two dissimilar mechanisms of action.

4.10 SUMMARY

The previous sections have described some of the preclinical hurdles and considerations when developing a relatively simple transdermal drug delivery device. The commercial, scale-up, manufacturing/fabrication, quality, safety, and efficacy issues that arise when clinical investigations and then marketing authorisation/NDA preparation and submission commences should not be underestimated. As such, relatively few active devices have gained regulatory approval compared to passive patches, and the success of these approved active transdermal delivery devices has been somewhat limited and is disappointing when the scale of dollar investment in these technologies is considered. Nevertheless, perhaps now is the time that these devices will come to the fore, with the recent advances in miniaturisation and electronics and the recovery from the recent financial crisis. However, as stated throughout this chapter, despite technological advances, it is important that the cost, design, manufacturing/fabrication, market, and end user (as well as the obvious safety, quality, efficacy requirements) all need to align to make the end product commercially viable. Perhaps the evolution of biological drugs will make the above approaches more compelling.

BIBLIOGRAPHY

Akomeah, F., Nazir, T., Martin, G.P., and Brown, M.B. (2004). Effect of heat on the percutaneous absorption and skin retention of three model penetrants. *Eur. J. Pharm. Sci.* 21(2–3): 337–345.

Allena, M.T. and Cullis, P.R. (2013). Liposomal drug delivery systems: from concept to clinical applications. *Adv. Drug. Deliv. Rev.* 65: 36–48.

Banga, A.K. (2011). Iontophoretic intradermal and transdermal drug delivery. In: *Transdermal and Intradermal Delivery of Therapeutic Agents: Application of Physical Technologies.* Boca Raton, FL: CRC Press, pp. 81–129.

Blank, I.H., Scheuplein, R.J., and Macfarlane, D.J. (1967). Mechanism of percutaneous absorption. *J. Invest. Dermatol.* 49(6): 582–589.

Burkoth, T.L., Bellhouse, B.J., Hewson, G., Longridge, D.J., Muddle, A.G., and Sarphie, D.F. (1999). Transdermal and transmucosal powdered drug delivery. *Crit. Rev. Ther. Drug Carrier Syst.* 16: 331–384.

Carrer, D.C., Higa, L.H., Tesoriero, M.V.D., Morilla, M.J., Roncaglia, D.I., and Romero, E.L. (2014). Structural features of ultradeformable archaeosomes for topical delivery of ovalbumin. *Colloids Surf. B Biointerfaces* 121: 281–289.

Cevc, G. and Blume, G. (1992). Lipid vesicles penetrate into intact skin owing to the transdermal osmotic gradient and hydration force. *Biochim. Biophys. Acta* 1104: 226–232.

Cevc, G. (1996). Transfersomes, liposomes and other lipid suspensions on the skin: permeation enhancement, vesicle penetration and transdermal drug delivery. *Crit. Rev. Ther. Drug Carrier Syst.* 13: 257–388.

Cevc, G., Blume, G., and Schatzlein, A. (1997). Transfersome-mediated transepidermal delivery improves the regio-specificity and biological activity of corticosteroids in vivo. *J. Control. Release* 45: 211–226.

Cevc, G. and Blume, G. (2001). New, highly efficient formulation of diclofenac for the topical, transdermal administration in ultradeformable drug carriers, Transfersomes. *Biochim. Biophys. Acta* 1514: 191–205.

Cevc, G., Blume, G., Schatzlein, A., Gebauer, D., and Paul A. (1996). The skin: a pathway for systemic treatment with patches and lipid-based carriers. *Adv. Drug. Deliv. Rev.* 18: 349–378.

Cevc, G. and Vierl, U. (2010). Nanotechnology and the transdermalroute: a state of the art review and critical appraisal. *J. Control. Release* 141: 277–299.

Cevc, G. (2012). Rational design of new product candidates: the next generation of highly deformable bilayer vesicles for noninvasive, targeted therapy. *J. Control. Release* 160: 135–146.

Chandel, A., Patil, V., Goya,l R., Dhamija, H., and Parashar, B. (2012). Ethosomes: a novel approach towards transdermal drug delivery. *Int. J. Pharm. Chem. Sci.* 1: 563–569.

Choi, M.J. and Maibach, H.I. (2005). Elastic vesicles as topical/transdermaldrug delivery system. *Int. J. Cosmet. Sci.* 27: 211–221.

Cummings, E.G. (1969). Temperature and concentration effects on penetration of N-octylamine through human skin in situ. *J. Invest. Dermatol.* 53(1): 64–70.

Donnelly, R.F., Garland, M.J., and Alkilani, A.Z. (2014). Microneedle-iontophoresis combinations for enhanced transdermal drug delivery. *Methods Mol. Biol.* 1141: 121–132.

El Maghraby, G.M.M., Williams, A.C., and Barry B.W. (1999). Skin delivery of estradiol from deformable and traditional liposomes: mechanistic studies. *J. Pharm. Pharmacol.* 51: 1123–1134.

Escobar-Chávez, J.J., Bonilla-Martinez, D., and Villegas-González, M.A. (2010). Sonophoresis: a valuable physical enhancer to increased transdermal drug delivery. In: Escobar-Chávez, J.J. (Ed.), *Current Technologies to Increase the Transdermal Delivery of Drugs.* Sharjah, U.A.E.: Bentham Science Publishers, pp. 53–77.

Escobar-Chávez, J.J., Bonilla-Martínez, D., Villegas-González, M.A., Molina-Trinidad, E., Casas-Alancaster, N., and Revilla-Vázquez, A.L. (2011). Microneedles: a valuable physical enhancer to increase transdermal drug delivery. *J. Clin. Pharm.* 51(7): 964–977.

Essa, E.A., Bonner, M.C., and Barry, B.W. (2002). Iontophoretic estradiol skin delivery and tritium exchange in ultradeformable liposomes. *Int. J. Pharm.* 240: 55–66.

Fritsch, W.C., Stoughton, R.B., and Stapelfeldt, A. (1963). The effect of temperature and humidity on the penetration of C14 acetylsalicylic acid in excised human skin. *J. Invest. Dermatol.* 41(5): 307–311.

Gan, L., Wang, J., Jiang, M., Bartlett, H., Ouyang, D., Eperjesi, F., Liu, J., and Gan, Y. 2013. Recent advances in topicalophthalmic drug delivery with lipid-based nanocarriers. *Drug Discov. Today* 18: 290–297.

Gonzalez-Rodrıgueza, M.L., Arroyo, C.M., Cozar-Bernal, M.J., Gonzalez-R., P.L., Leon, J.M., Calle, J.M., Canca, D., and Rabasco, A.M. (2016). Deformability properties of timolol-loaded transfersomes based on the extrusion mechanism. Statistical optimization of the process. *Drug Dev. Ind. Pharm.* 42 (10): 1683–1694.

Gupta, A., Aggarwal, G., Singla, S., and Arora, R. (2012). Transfersomes: a novel vesicular carrier for enhanced transdermal delivery of sertraline: development, characterization and performance evaluation. *Sci. Pharm.* 80: 1061–1080.

Guy, R.H. (1998). Iontophoresis – recent developments. *J. Pharm. Pharmacol.* 50: 371–374.

Haedersdal, M., Erlendsson, A.M., Paasch, U., and Anderson, R.R. (2016). Translational medicine in the field of ablative fractional laser (AFXL)-assisted drug delivery: a critical review from basics to current clinical status. *J. Am. Acad. Dermatol.* 74: 981–1004.

Haensler, J., Verdelet, C., Sanchez, V., Girerd-Chambaz, Y., Bonnin, A., Trannoy, E., Krishnan, S., and Meulien, P. (1999). Intradermal DNA immunization by using jet-injectors in mice and monkeys. *Vaccine* 17: 628–638.

Henry, S., McAllister, D.V., Allen, M.G., and Prausnitz, M.R. (1998). Microfabricated microneedles: a novel approach to transdermal drug delivery. *J. Pharm. Sci.* 87: 922–925.

Hofland, H.E.J., van der Geest, R., Bodde, H.E., Junginger, H.E., and Bouwstra, J.A. (1994). Estradiol permeation from non-ionic surfactant vesicles through human stratum corneum in vitro. *Pharm. Res.* 11: 659–664.

Honzak, L. and Sentjure, M. (2000). Development of liposome encapsulated clindamycin for treatment of acne vulgaris. *Eur. J. Physiol.* 440: R44–R45.

Hu Z., Niemiec S.M., Ramachandran C., Wallach D.F.H., and Weiner N. (1994). Topical delivery of cyclosporine-A from non-ionic liposomal systems – an in vivo in vitro correlation study using hairless mouse skin. *STP Pharma Sci.* 4: 466–469.

Hua, S. (2015). Lipid-based nano-delivery systems for skin delivery of drugs and bioactives. *Front. Pharmacol.* 8: 1–5.

Hughes, P.J., Freeman, M.K., and Wensel, T.M. (2013). Appropriate use of transdermal drug delivery systems. *J. Nurs. Educ. Pract.* 3: 129–138.

Immordino, M.L, Dosio, F., and Cattel, L. (2006). Stealth liposomes: review of the basic science, rationale, and clinical applications, existing and potential. *Int. J. Nanomed.* 1: 297–315.

Jacques, S.L., McAuliffe, D.J., Blank, I.H., and Parrish, J.A. (1987). Controlled removal of human stratum corneum by pulsed laser. *J. Invest. Dermatol.* 88: 88–93.

Jain, S. and Jain, P. (2003). Transferosomes: a novel vesicular carrier for enhanced transdermal delivery: development, characterization and performance evaluation. *Drug Dev. Ind. Pharm.* 29: 1013–1026.

Jain, S., Patel, N., Shah, M.K., Khatri, P., and Vora, N. (2016). Recent advances in lipid-based vesicles and particulate carriers for topical and transdermal application. *J. Pharm. Sci.* 116: 1–23.

Johnson, M.E., Mitragotri, S., Patel, A., Blankschtein, D., and Langer, R. (1996). Synergistic effects of chemical enhancers and therapeutic ultrasound on transdermal drug delivery. *J. Pharm. Sci.* 85: 670–679.

Kankkunen, T., Sulkava, R., Vuorio, M., Kontturi, K., and Hirvonen, J. (2002). Transdermal iontophoresis of tacrine in vivo. *Pharm. Res.* 19: 705–708.

Kaushik, S., Hord, A.H., Denson, D.D., McAllister, D.V., Smitra, S., Allen, M.G., and Prausnitz, M.R. (2001). Lack of pain associated with microfabricated microneedles. *Anesth. Analg.* 92: 502–504.

Kost, J., Pliquett, U., Mitragotri, S., Yamamoto, A., Langer, R., and Weaver, J. (1996). Synergistic effects of electric field and ultrasound on transdermal transport. *Pharm. Res.* 13: 633–638.

Kreuter, J. (1994). Nanoparticles. In Swarbrick, J., Boylan, J.C. (Eds.), *Encyclopedia of Pharmaceutical Technology*, Marcel Dekker, Inc, New York, NY, pp. 165–290.

Lauterbach, A. and Müller-Goymann, C.C. (2015). Applications and limitations of lipid nanoparticles in dermal and transdermal drug delivery via the follicular route. *Eur. J. Pharm. Biopharm.* 97: 152–163.

Lasic, D.D. (1998). Novel applications of liposomes. *Trends Biotechnol.* 16: 307–321.

Lee, S., Kollias, N., McAuliffe, D.J., Flotte, T.J., and Doukas, A.G. (1999). Topical delivery in humans with a single photomechanical wave. *Pharm. Res.* 16: 1717–1721.

Lee, S., McAuliffe, D.J., Flotte, T.J., Kollias, N., and Doukas, A.G. (2001b). Photomechanical transdermal delivery: the effect of laser confinement. *Lasers Surg. Med.* 28: 344–347.

Lee, S., McAuliffe, D.J., Flotte, T.J., Kollias, N., and Doukas, A.G. (2001c). Permeabilization and recovery of the stratum corneum in vivo: the synergy of photomechanical waves and sodium lauryl sulfate. *Lasers Surg. Med.* 29: 145–150.

Lee, W.R., Shen, S.C., Lai, H.H., Hu, C.H., and Fang, J.Y. (2001). Transdermal drug delivery enhanced and controlled by erbium: YAG laser: a comparative study of lipophilic and hydrophilic drugs. *J. Control. Release* 75: 155–166.

Lee, H., Song, C., Baik, S., Kima, D., and Hyeon, T., Kim D-H (2018). Device-assisted transdermal drug delivery. *Adv. Drug Deliv. Rev.* 127: 35–45.

Lieb, L.M., Ramachandran, C., Egbaria, K., and Weiner, N. (1992). Topical delivery enhancement with multilamellar liposomes into pilosebaceous units: I. In vitro evaluation using fluorescent techniques with hamster ear model. *J. Invest. Dermatol.* 99: 108–113.

McAllister, D.V., Allen, M.G., and Prausnitz, M.R. (2000). Microfabricated microneedles for gene and drug delivery. *Annu. Rev. Biomed. Eng.* 2: 289–313.

McAuley, W.J. and Caserta, F. (2015). Film-forming and heated systems. In: Donnelly, R.F. and Singh, T.R.R. (Eds.), *Novel Delivery Systems for Transdermal and Intradermal Drug Delivery*. Chichester, U.K.: John Wiley & Sons, Ltd, pp. 97–124.

Michel, C., Purmann, T., Mentrup, E., Seiller, E., and Kreuter, J. (1992). Effect of liposomes on percutaneous penetration of lipophilic materials. *Int. J. Pharm.* 84(2): 93–105.

Mitragotri, S. (2000). Synergistic effect of enhancers for transdermal drug delivery. *Pharm. Res.* 17: 1354–1359.

Mitragotri, S., Edwards, D., Blankschtein, D., and Langer, R. (1995a). A mechanistic study of ultrasonically enhanced transdermal drug delivery. *J. Pharm. Sci.* 84: 697–706.

Mitragotri, S., Blankschtein, D., and Langer, R. (1995b). Ultrasound-mediated transdermal protein delivery. *Science* 269: 850–853.

Mitragotri, S., Blankschtein, D., and Langer, R. (1996). Transdermal drug delivery using low-frequency sonophoresis. *Pharm. Res.* 13: 411–420.

Moritz, A.R. and Henriques, F.C. (1947). Studies of thermal injury. II. The relative importance of time and surface temperature in the causation of cutaneous burns. *Am. J. Pathol.* 23(5): 695–720.

Müller, R.H., Mäder, K., and Gohla, S. (2000). Solid lipid nanoparticles (SLN) for controlled-drug delivery – a review of the state of the art. *Eur. J. Pharm. Biopharm.* 50: 161–177.

Murthy, S.N. (1999). Magnetophoresis: an approach to enhance transdermal drug diffusion. *Pharmazie* 54: 377–379.

Nadler, S.F., Steiner, D.J., Erasala, G.N., Hengehold, D.A., Hinkle, R.T., Beth Goodale M., and Weingand, K.W. (2002). Continuous low-level heat wrap therapy provides more efficacy than Ibuprofen and acetaminophen for acute low back pain. *Spine* 27(10): 1012–1017.

Nadler, S.F., Steiner, D.J., Petty, S.R., Erasala, G.N., Hengehold, D.A., and Weingand, K.W. (2003). Overnight use of continuous low-level heatwrap therapy for relief of low back pain. *Arch. Phys. Med. Rehabil.* 84(3): 335–342.

Nelson, J.S., McCullough, J.L., Glenn, T.C., Wright, W.H., Liaw, L.H., and Jacques, S.L. (1991). Mid-infrared laser ablation of stratum corneum enhances in vitro percutaneous transport of drugs. *J. Invest. Dermatol.* 97: 874–879.

New, R.C.C. (1990). *Liposomes: A Practical Approach*. Oxford: Oxford University Press.

Nounou, M.I., El-Khordagui, L.K., Khalafallah, N.A., and Khalil, S.A. (2008). Liposomal formulation for dermal and transdermal drug delivery: past, present and future. *Recent Pat. Drug Deliv. Formul.* 2: 9–18.

Ogiso, T., Yamaguchi, T., Iwaki, M., Tanino, T., and Miyake, Y. (2001). Effect of positively and negatively charged liposomes on skin permeation of drugs. *J. Drug Target.* 9: 49–61.

Ogura, M., Paliwal, S., and Mitragotri, S. (2008). Low-frequency sonophoresis: current status and future prospects. *Adv. Drug Deliv. Rev.* 60(10): 1218–1223.

Olatunji, O., Al-Qallaf, B., and Das, D.B. (2010). Transdermal drug delivery using microneedles. In: Escobar-Chávez, J.J. (Ed.), *Current Technologies to Increase the Transdermal Delivery of Drugs*. Sharjah: Bentham Science Publishers, pp. 96–119.

Oliveira, G., Leverett, J.C., Emamzadeh, M., and Lane, M.E. (2014). The effects of heat on skin barrier function and in vivo dermal absorption. *Int. J. Pharm.* 464(1–2): 145–151.

Pahade, A, Jadhav, V.M., and Kadam, V.J. (2010). Sonophoresis: an overview. *Int. J. Pharm. Sci. Rev. Res.* 3(2): 24–32.

Patel, V.B., Misra, A., and Marfatia, Y.S. (2000). Topical liposomal gel of tretinoin for the treatment of acne: research and clinical implications. *Pharm. Dev. Tech.* 5: 455–464.

Paudel, K.S., Milewski, M., Swadley, C.L., Brogden, N.K., Ghosh, P., and Stinchcomb, A.L. (2010). Challenges and opportunities in dermal/transdermal delivery. *Ther. Deliv.* 1: 109–131.

Paul, A., Cevc, G., and Bachhawat, B.K. (1995). Transdermal immunization with large proteins by means of ultradeformable drug carriers. *Eur. J. Immunol.* 25: 3521–3524.

Pawar, K.R. and Babu, R.J. (2014). Lipid materials for topical and transdermal delivery of nanoemulsions. *Crit. Rev. Ther. Drug Carrier Syst.* 31: 429–458.

Perumal, O., Murthy, S., and Kalia, Y. (2013). Turning theory into practice: the development of modern transdermal drug delivery systems and future trends. *Skin Pharm. Physiol.* 26: 331–342.

Pikal, M.J. and Shah, S. (1990). Transport mechanisms in iontophoresis. II. Electroosmotic flow and transference number measurements for hairless mouse skin. *Pharm. Res.* 7: 213–221.

Pliquett, E.F. and Gusbeth, C.A. (2000). Perturbation of human skin due to application of high voltage. *Bioelectrochemistry* 51: 41–51.

Potts, R.O., Tamada, J.A., and Tierney, M.J. (2002). Glucose monitoring by reverse iontophoresis. *Diabetes-Metab. Res. Rev.* 18: S49–S53.

Prausnitz, M.R. (1999). A practical assessment of transdermal drug delivery by skin electroporation. *Adv. Drug Deliv. Rev.* 35: 61–76.

Prausnitz, M.R., Bose, V.G., Langer, R., and Weaver, J.C. (1993). Electroporation of mammalian skin: a mechanism to enhance transdermal drug delivery. *Proc. Natl. Acad. Sci. USA* 90: 10504–10508.

Prausnitz, M.R. and Langer, R. (2008). Transdermal drug delivery. *Nat. Biotechnol.* 26: 1261–1268.

Prausnitz, M.R., Mikszta, J.A., Cormier, M., and Andrianov, A.K. (2009). Microneedle-based vaccines. *Curr. Top. Microbiol. Immunol.* 333: 369–393.

Quinn, H.L., Courtenay, A.J., Kearney, M.-C., and Donnelly, R.F. (2015). Microneedle technology. In: Donnelly, R.F. and Singh, T.R.R. (Eds.), *Novel Delivery Systems for Transdermal and Intradermal Drug Delivery*. Chichester, UK: John Wiley & Sons, Ltd, pp. 179–208.

Quinlan, N.J., Kendall, M.A.F., Bellhouse, B.J. and Ainsworth, R.W. (2001). Investigations of gas and particle dynamics in first generation needle-free drug delivery devices. *Shock Waves* 10: 395–404.

Rastogi, S.K. and Singh, J. (2002). Transepidermal transport enhancement of insulin by lipid extraction and iontophoresis. *Pharm. Res.* 19: 427–433.

Rai, S., Pandey, V., and Rai, G. (2017). Transfersomes as versatile and flexible nano-vesicular carriers in skin cancer therapy: the state of the art. *Nano Rev. Exp.* 8: 1–17.

Roberts, M.S., Mohammed, Y., Pastore, M.N., Namjoshi, S., Yousef, S., Alinaghi, A., Haridass, I.N., Abd, E., Leite-Silva, V.R., Benson, H.A.E., and Grice, J.E. (2017). Topical and cutaneous delivery using nanosystems. *J. Control. Release* 247: 86–105.

Santi, P. and Guy, R.H. (1996). Reverse iontophoresis – parameters determining electroosmotic flow: 1. pH and ionic strength. *J. Control. Release* 38: 159–165.

Sarphie, D.F., Johnson, B., Cormier, M., Burkoth, T.L., and Bellhouse, B.J. (1997). Bioavailability following transdermal powdered delivery (TPD) of radiolabelled inulin to hairless guinea pigs. *J. Control. Release* 47: 61–69.

Sawyer, J., Febbraro, S., Masud, S., Ashburn, M.A., and Campbell, J.C. (2009). Heated lidocaine/tetracaine patch (SyneraTM, RapydanTM) compared with lidocaine/prilocaine cream (EMLA®) for topical anaesthesia before vascular access. *Br. J. Anaesth.* 102(2): 210–215.

Sercombe, L., Veerati, T., Moheimani, F., Wu, S.Y., Sood, A.K., and Hua, S. (2015). Advances and challenges of liposome assisted drug delivery. *Front. Pharmacol.* 6: 286.

Singh, S., and Singh, J. (1993). Transdermal drug delivery by passive diffusion and iontophoresis: a review. *Med. Res. Rev.* 13(5): 569–621.

Shahzad, Y., Louw, R., Gerber, M., and du Plessis, J. (2015). Breaching the skin barrier through temperature modulations. *J. Control. Release* 202: 1–13.

Smith, N.B. (2007). Perspectives on transdermal ultrasound mediated drug delivery. *Int. J. Nanomed.* 2(4): 585–594.

Smyth, H.D.C., Becket, C., and Mehta, S. (2002). Effect of permeation enhancer pre-treatment on the iontophoresis of luteinizing hormone releasing hormone (LHRH) through human epidermal membrane (HEM). *J. Pharm. Sci.* 91: 1296–1307.

Stanley, T., Hull, W., and Rigby, L. (2001). Transdermal drug patch with attached pocket for controlled heating device. US6488959B2. United States Patent, United States.

Sreeraj, S.R., Bharati, B., and Ipseeta, R. (2015). A review on ultrasound parameters and methods of application in transdermal drug delivery. *Int. J. Health Sci. Res.* 5: 476–485.

Tamada, J.A., Bohannon, N.J.V., and Potts, R.O. (1995). Measurement of glucose in diabetic subjects using non-invasive transdermal extraction. *Nat. Med.* 1: 1198–1201.

Terahara, T., Mitragotri, S., Kost, J., and Langer, R. (2002). Dependence of low-frequency sonophoresis on ultrasound parameters; distance of the horn and intensity. *Int. J. Pharm.* 235: 35–42.

Tierney, M.J., Tamada, J.A., Potts, R.O., Jovanovic, L., and Garg, S. (2001). Clinical evaluation of the GlucoWatch®biographer: a continual, non-invasive glucose monitor for patients with diabetes. *Biosens. Bioelectron.* 16: 621–629.

Touitou, E., Alkabes, M., Dayan, N., and Eliaz, M. (1997). Ethosomes: novel vesicular carriers for enhanced skin delivery. *Pharm. Res.* 14: S305–306.

Touitou, E., Dayan, N., Bergelson, L., Godin, B., and Eliaz, M. (2000). Ethosomes – novel vesicular carriers for enhanced delivery: characterisation and skin penetration properties. *J. Control. Release* 65: 403–418.

Touitou, E., Godin, B., and Weiss, C. (2000). Enhanced delivery of drugs into and across the skin by ethosomal carriers. *Drug Dev. Res.* 50: 406–415.

Uchegbu, I.F. and Florence, A.T. (1995). Nonionic surfactant vesicles (niosomes) – physical and pharmaceutical chemistry. *Adv. Colloid Interface Sci.* 58: 1–55.

Uchegbu, I.F. and Vyas, S.P. (1998). Non-ionic surfactant based vesicles (niosomes) in drug delivery. *Int. J. Pharm.* 172: 33–70.

van Hal, D.A., Jeremiasse, E., de Vringer, T., Junginger, H.E., and Bouwstra, J.A. (1996). Encapsulation of lidocaine base and hydrochloride into non-ionic surfactant vesicles (NSVs) and diffusion through human stratum corneum in vitro. *Eur. J. Pharm. Sci.* 4: 147–157.

Vemuri, S. and Rhodes, C.T. (1995). Preparation and characterization of liposomes as therapeutic delivery systems. *Pharm. Acta Helv.* 70: 95–111.

Weiner, N., Williams, N., Birch, G., Ramachandran, C., Shipman, C.J.R. and Flynn, G.L. (1989). Topical delivery of liposomally encapsulated interferon evaluated in cutaneous herpes guinea pig model. *Antimicrob. Agents Chemother.* 33: 1217–1221.

Wood, D.G., Brown, M.B. and Jones, S.A. (2012). Understanding heat facilitated drug transport across human epidermis. *Eur. J. Pharm. Biopharm.* 81(3): 642–649.

Wood, D.G., Brown, M.B., Jones, S.A., and Murnane, D. (2011). Characterization of latent heat-releasing phase change materials for dermal therapies. *J. Phys. Chem. C* 115(16): 8369–8375.

Wu, Q.H., Liang, W.Q., Bao, J.L., and Ping, Q.N. (2000). Enhanced transdermal delivery of tetracaine by electroporation. *Int. J. Pharm.* 202: 121–124.

Yeoh, T. (2012). Current landscape and trends in transdermal drug delivery systems. *Ther. Deliv.* 3: 295–297.

Zewert, T.E., Pliquett, U.F., Vanbever, R., Langer, R., and Weaver, J.C. (1999). Creation of transdermal pathways for macromolecule transport by skin electroporation and a low toxicity, pathway-enlarging molecule. *Bioelectrochem. Bioenerg.* 49: 11–20.

Zharov, V.P. and Laytshev, A.S. (1998). Biotransport: heat and mass transfer in living systems. *Ann. NY Acad. Sci.* 858: 66–73.

Zylberberg, C. and Matosevic, S. (2016). Pharmaceutical liposomal drug delivery: a review of new delivery systems and a look at the regulatory landscape. *Drug Deliv.* 23(9): 3319–3329.

5 Topical and Transdermal Formulation Development

5.1 INTRODUCTION

When a formulation scientist starts the long and often painful process of developing a topical or transdermal formulation, there are numerous issues that need to be considered. However, it should always be remembered that it is not a drug that you give to a patient but a drug product (i.e., a medicine), and the pharmaceutical history is littered with examples of drugs that could have been the next "magic bullet" or turned into the next blockbuster if only a formulation could have been developed to deliver the molecule safely and efficaciously to their pathological site in a cost-effective manner. Such problems are exacerbated even further in dermal drug delivery, in that patients care about, and often have a choice in, what they apply to the skin. As such, the patient or consumer should often be at the forefront of the thoughts of a formulation scientist. The dermal products developed many years ago that were greasy, with poor odour, and that stained clothes are no longer acceptable; cosmetics and aesthetics of the final product are *almost* as important (some brand managers would argue that this should read "*more* important") as the product's efficacy. A good example of this is the relatively recent development of topical foam products which may add no real benefit in terms of drug delivery but provide the consumer with an alternative that is easy to apply cosmetically and is just "different" to the classic semi-solids such as creams and ointments that the consumer is used to.

A plethora of possibilities exist when preparing formulations for topical or transdermal therapy. Many elegant and novel drug delivery systems are available for formulating skin preparations, as well as several where extravagant claims may be unfounded. It is not the intention to deal with all of these formulations but rather to describe the principal formulations used to effectively deliver medicaments to, and across, the skin, with more emphasis on the former.

5.2 A TARGET PRODUCT PROFILE

In general, the selection of a vehicle for topical application is influenced by the physicochemical properties of the drug, the disease to which it is applied, and the patient who will use it (however, there are other considerations – see Section 4.2). Thus, in any resultant formulation, the stability and compatibility of the excipients with the drugs and with themselves must be considered, whilst ensuring that the preparation is cosmetically acceptable with a good skin-feel, texture, and fragrance. A schematic

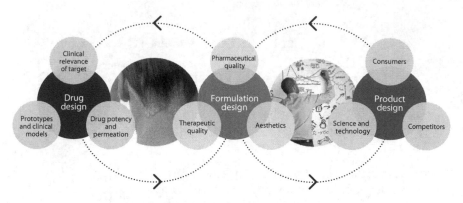

FIGURE 5.1   **(See color insert.)** Common considerations for topical product development.

of what needs to be considered when establishing a profile of the intended product is provided in Figure 5.1.

For transdermal delivery where systemic drug delivery is required, most of the above considerations apply but in different ways. For example, the appearance and acceptability (aesthetics) of the patch need to be considered, as it still needs to be applied and worn, but the disease or condition being treated generally has a lesser influence than with dermal application; achieving the required drug plasma levels over the lifetime of the patch is a greater concern. Additionally, the drug payload left in the patch also needs to be thought about, especially for those drugs that may be illicitly abused.

As can be seen, when building up an overarching product "wish list", there needs to be input from various stakeholders, including a medicinal chemist (sometimes with a computational modeller), an analyst, a formulator, a toxicologist, a clinician, and representation from the regulatory, quality, manufacturing, marketing, and/or commercial departments. Getting written agreement is critical at this stage to maximise the chances of success and avoid wasting money on the development of a product that will never reach the market. Generally, such a document is called a Target Product Profile (TPP) and is often an evolving document as things progress. Examples of what may be considered for a TPP are provided in Figure 5.2, but obviously the relative importance of each criterion depends upon the type of product being developed. A

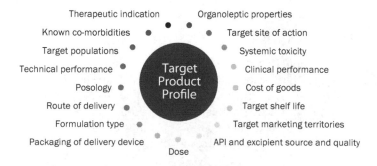

FIGURE 5.2   **(See color insert.)** Considerations for a Target Product Profile.

TPP can often help in the production of a Quality Target Product Profile (QTPP), the latter often being a subset of the former, described in detail in Section 5.4.

5.3 THE PHARMACEUTICAL DEVELOPMENT PROCESS

An overview of a generic formulation development process, beginning from preformulation development up to identification of the final lead formulation candidate, is summarised in the flowchart shown in Figure 5.3. With this in mind, the remainder of this chapter provides an overview of some of the steps and hurdles that a formulation scientist should work through to develop a product that will be optimised for the drug, formulation, disease, and consumer.

5.4 QUALITY BY DESIGN

5.4.1 THE PRINCIPLES OF QUALITY BY DESIGN IN PRODUCT DEVELOPMENT

The principles of Quality by Design (QbD) were first described in the 1950s. These highlighted that quality must be designed into a product using a process-understanding approach during the manufacturing process rather than by using a Quality by Testing (QbT) system, which is an unbending process with its bound specifications for its manufactured batches. More recently, such an approach has been pushed back in the development process to also cover preformulation and formulation development. As such, the U.S. Food and Drug Administration (FDA) encourages a risk-based QbD approach in drug product development (companies are expected to incorporate basic QbD elements in abbreviated new drug application [ANDA] product filings) and transition to more complete QbD filings as industry and regulatory agencies synchronise knowledge gained from successful and unsuccessful experiences.

According to the FDA and the guidelines of the International Conference on Harmonisation (ICH) Q8(R2), pharmaceutical QbD can be defined as a systematic approach to product development that aims to ensure the quality of pharmaceutical products by employing statistical, analytical, and risk management methodology during design, development, and manufacturing. The objective is to identify any Critical Process Parameters (CPPs) and Critical Material Attributes (CMAs) that should be monitored and/or controlled to achieve the best quality product.

The regulatory framework for Pharmaceutical QbD follows the ICH guidelines Q8 (R2) (Pharmaceutical Development), Q9 (Quality Risk Management), and Q10 (Pharmaceutical Quality System). Additionally, the FDA and the European Medicines Agency (EMA) have issued the ICH Q1WG on Q8, Q9, and Q10 Questions and Answers; the ICH Q8/Q9/Q10 Points to Consider; and the ICH Q11 (Development and Manufacture of Drug Substance), which provide more specific guidelines with respect to QbD in the pharmaceutical industry.

The ICH Q8 (R2) guideline for pharmaceutical development comprises all the elements required for a QbD approach. The different stages defined in this document are as follows:

1. Define an objective by determining the Quality Product Profile (QPP).
2. Determine Critical Quality Attributes (CQAs) by a criticality assessment.

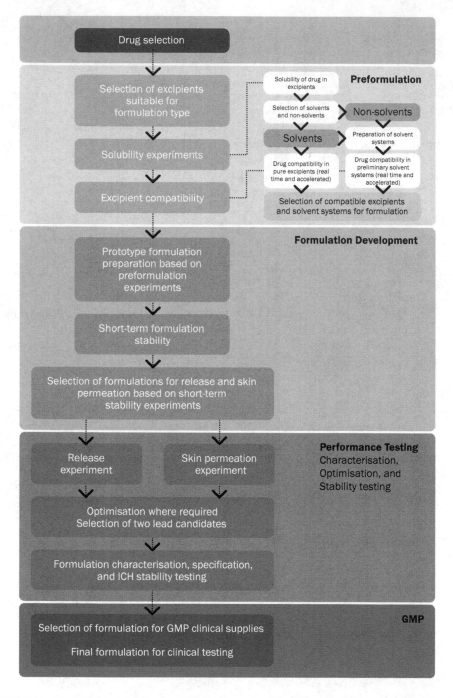

FIGURE 5.3 (See color insert.) Flowchart summarising key events of a typical topical semi-solid formulation development program.

3. Perform a risk assessment in order to link raw Material Attributes (MAs) and Process Parameters (PPs) to CQAs.
4. Develop a Design Space (DS) to identify a Control Space (CS) where the Design of Experiment (DoE) can be defined.
5. Design and implement a control strategy to ensure that CQAs are met.
6. Continual improvement during the product lifecycle.

Some of these are described in greater detail below.

5.4.2 QUALITY TARGET PRODUCT PROFILE AND CRITICAL QUALITY ATTRIBUTES

The Quality Target Product Profile (QTPP) defines the design and development of the desired pharmaceutical product and is a prospective summary of the quality characteristics of a drug product that ideally will be achieved to ensure the desired quality, taking into account the safety and efficacy of the drug product. As such this is often a subset of the Target Product Profile previously discussed. The production of a QTPP leads to the identification of Critical Quality Attributes (CQAs). ICH Q8(R2) defines a CQA as "a property or characteristic that when controlled within a defined limit, range, or distribution ensures the desired product quality". CQAs are normally associated with the API, excipients, in process materials (intermediates), and drug product. With the aid of quality risk management (ICH Q9) and statistical design of experiments, Critical Material Attributes of the drug, excipients, and product, including:

- Purity
- Particle size and distribution
- Molecular weight and/or polydispersity
- Solid state properties
- Viscosity, rheology, and microstructure of material
- Polymorphic state
- Crystalline habit

and Critical Processing Parameters (CPPs) such as:

- Order of addition
- Rate and mechanism of addition
- pH and temperature
- Homogenisation/stirring rate and speed
- Cooling rate and speed

can be identified that impact upon the CQAs and thus the quality of the product, such as:

- The phase states and the arrangement of matter (microstructure)
- Drug diffusion within the dosage form

- Drug stability within the dosage form
- Drug release and partitioning from the dosage form into the stratum corneum
- Alteration of skin structure and chemistry
- Drug diffusion within the skin itself
- Drug delivery and bioavailability at the target site
- Skin (de)hydration, irritation, or damage
- Metamorphosis of the dosage form on the skin

The final step is to establish a design space. ICH Q8 (R2) defines a design space as the "multidimensional combination and interaction of input variables (e.g., material attributes) and processing parameters that have been demonstrated to provide the assurance of quality".

5.4.3 Risk Assessment (ICH Q9)

The ICH Q9 defines risk assessment as the combination of the probability of occurrence and the severity of the identified risk. Therefore, a risk assessment on a pharmaceutical product determines the effect of input variables on the process. Some methods for risk assessment described by the ICH Q9 are: Failure Mode Effects Analysis (FMEA); Failure Mode, Effects, and Criticality Analysis (FMECA); basic risk management facilitation (flowcharts, check sheets); risk ranking and filtering; supporting statistical tools; Ishikawa diagrams; and "what if" analysis (ICH Q8[R2], 2009). A quality risk management guideline ICH Q9 recognises that the development, manufacture, and use of a pharmaceutical product is associated with a degree of risk for the consumer/patient. However, the risk–quality ratio must be considered, and must favour therapeutic effectiveness and safety.

5.4.4 Design Space (DS) and Development of the Design of Experiment

Experimental design or design space is defined as the multidimensional combination and interaction of material attributes and process parameters that have been demonstrated to provide assurance of quality. A DS accounts for the interaction between factors, a Multi-Factorial Design (MFD) affecting product quality. However, it is important to recognise and avoid confounding factors, as this will not allow clear boundaries to be defined within the experimental design. The DS is developed based on current or previous experimental data, literature reviews, and/or product experience. A DS provides a clear material and process understanding; thus, operating within its limits is not considered a change. However, if any changes are made outside the established limits within the DS, regulatory guidance must be sought. As such, a defined DS is advantageous in terms of anticipating issues that may arise during manufacture and planning in advance how to control the process. Once the DS has been defined, a control space can be determined. To best identify the control space, a Design of Experiments is developed as a tool that systematically manipulates factors according to the pre-defined DS. Additionally, a DoE demonstrates the relationships between input factors and output responses. As opposed to the traditional approach of One Factor At a Time (OFAT), a DoE is based on a Multi-Factorial Design (MFD) where it is possible to observe how factors jointly influence the output responses.

5.5   TOPICAL (DERMAL) FORMULATION OPTIONS

Topical dosage forms have been generally classified as liquids, semi-solids, and solids, and typical examples are summarised in Figure 5.4.

5.5.1   LIQUID FORMULATIONS

Liquid formulations can be simple single-phase solutions, either aqueous, or prepared from a solvent, an oil, or from miscible co-solvents. The preparations can thus be, for example, a soak (or bath) or paint. Liquid formulations can also be two-phase systems, such as with thin oil-in-water (o/w) or water-in-oil (w/o) emulsions (lotions) or as with a suspension typically of powder in an aqueous solution, or can be multi-phase when using more complex oil-in-water-in-oil (o/w/o) or water-in-oil-in-water (w/o/w) systems. The designation of an emulsion between a "liquid" and a "semi-solid" is somewhat arbitrary, but emulsions are most widely used in creams.

Although some commercial single-phase liquid preparations for topical application are available, including, for example, lotions of carbaryl (carbaril) and malathion to treat lice or solutions of cetrimide or chlorhexidine for skin disinfection, simple liquid preparations are seldom used for topical and transdermal delivery. Generally, such liquid systems have a relatively poor residence time on the skin and thus delivery is limited to a short timeframe.

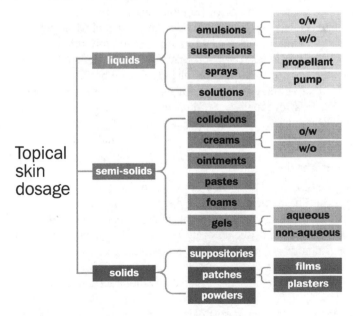

FIGURE 5.4   Summary of typical topical dosage forms.

Two-phase or multi-phase liquid systems are rather more widely used to deliver medicines to, and through, the skin. Lotions containing an aqueous suspension cool the skin as the water evaporates from the tissue surface, an effect that is enhanced if alcohol is present in the formulation; alcohol-based lotions are not, however, suitable for broken skin. Either formulated as a single-phase lotion with the drug dissolved or as a two-phase system, such as a shake lotion where an insoluble powder is incorporated (for example, calamine lotion), evaporation of the vehicle deposits a film of the drug as a powder onto the tissue surface. Depositing a powder, or a thin film, onto the skin surface improves residence time and can be valuable for treating large convoluted tissue areas, although a deposited powder must then undergo a dissolution step prior to penetration into the stratum corneum. Delivery can occur during the drying phase of a lotion or solution applied to the skin surface. Indeed, on drying a solution, it is feasible that drug delivery will be enhanced through supersaturation: as the solvent is lost from the system, the permeant may reach a metastable state within the vehicle where its solubility exceeds its equilibrium solubility for a short period of time with a consequent increase in diffusional driving force and hence increasing drug delivery (see Chapter 3, Section 3.4.4). With a suspension, excess powder present in the formulation provides sites for crystallisation, and so the generation of a metastable solution of drug in excess of its solubility is unlikely.

5.5.2 Semi-Solid Formulations

The vast majority of topically applied preparations are semi-solids; they have good residence on the skin and can thus be used to deliver therapeutic agents over a period of time. Further, there are numerous options available to the formulator in preparing semi-solids. However, the classification of such topical dosage forms is often poorly defined and ambiguous depending on the literature referenced. For example, the European Pharmacopeia (EP) and British Pharmacopeia (BP) define ointments as "single-phase basis in which solids or liquids may be dispersed" and creams as "multiphase preparations consisting of a lipophilic phase and an aqueous phase", whilst the U.S. Pharmacopeia (USP) and the U.S. Food and Drug Administration (U.S. FDA) define ointments and creams as "a semisolid dosage form containing one or more drug substance dissolved or dispersed in a suitable base".

5.5.2.1 Ointments

An ointment can be defined as a greasy or fatty semi-solid preparation intended for application to the skin. The medicament may be dissolved in the vehicle or it may be present as a powder, usually micro-crystalline. Various ointment bases are available, but in general terms they are usually occlusive and so are suitable for use on dry lesions; non-medicated ointments are valuable as emollients in dry and eczematous disorders. Additionally, ointments may contain excipients such cetostearyl alcohol or silicones (polydimethylsiloxane oil or a dimethicone) to improve the spreadability of the formulation.

Hydrocarbon bases, such as soft paraffin or combinations of soft, liquid, and hard paraffins, are commonly used. These bases are anhydrous and form an occlusive layer on the skin surface, thus are very useful in their own right as emollients in dry scaling conditions. The hydrocarbon base components do not permeate through intact skin to any great extent and their use as drug delivery systems is limited due to the relatively poor solubility of most drugs in the base. Occlusion of the skin surface and the consequent increased hydration of the tissue would facilitate permeation of a therapeutic agent from a hydrocarbon ointment, as would the broken skin where these formulations are usually applied.

Absorption bases contain an emulsifying agent that will allow the formulation to soak up water or aqueous secretions whilst retaining a semi-solid consistency. The absorption base can generate a water-in-oil system when combining, for example, paraffins with polyhydric alcohols such as sorbitan monooleate. These bases can absorb around 15% water whilst remaining semi-solid, and provide some occlusion of the stratum corneum, suppressing moisture loss from the tissue. Thus, absorption base ointments also hydrate the stratum corneum and may be left in contact with the tissue for prolonged periods of time. Components traditionally used in absorption base ointments, such as wool fats and wool alcohols or purified lanolins have largely been superseded, as allergic reactions to these ingredients have been reported.

Emulsifying bases are somewhat similar to absorption bases but can form in oil-in-water systems, for example, using a mixture of paraffins with cetostearyl alcohol and a surface-active agent (e.g., sodium lauryl sulphate or cetrimide). The emulsifying agents thus generate a water-miscible ointment (i.e., they are self-emulsifying) which allows it to be readily washed from the skin, in contrast to the hydrocarbon bases. Differing bases can be prepared and are classified by the ionic nature of the emulsifying agent. Anionic emulsifying bases obviously contain an anionic emulsifying agent such as emulsifying wax, a mixture of cetostearyl alcohol and sodium lauryl sulphate. This is the agent that is found in Emulsifying Ointment BP, comprising liquid paraffin (20%), white soft paraffin (50%), and emulsifying wax (30%). Clearly, an anionic ointment is incompatible with a cationic therapeutic agent, as the structure of the base would be modified. Cationic emulsifying ointments containing, for example, cetrimide as the emulsifying agent are more suitable for use with cationic drugs and non-ionic emulsifying bases (such as using cetomacrogol as the emulsifier) can also be used with cationic medicaments. Since the emulsifying bases contain a surfactant, there exists potential for permeation enhancement from these bases, although as described earlier (Chapter 3, Section 3.2.2.7), surfactants are relatively poor permeation promoters. However, the surfactant can help to solubilise the therapeutic agent and to wet the skin surface.

Water-soluble bases contain mixtures of water-soluble high and low molecular weight polyethylene glycols (macrogols). These ethylene glycol polymers are analogous to the paraffins in that they range from mobile liquids to hard waxes and hence can be blended to form an ointment with the desired properties. Water-soluble bases have several important advantages over other ointment bases; they mix readily with skin secretions, they are chemically very stable, they soften at skin temperatures allowing them to spread easily (depending on the polymer composition), and they can be washed from the skin without difficulty. However, they do lose their semi-solid consistency if around 10% water is taken into the ointment, and they are incompatible with several classes of compounds including phenols and penicillin.

As can be seen from the above, many ointments are prepared from mixtures of hydrocarbons, such as paraffins. It is important to remember that various grades and qualities of these materials are available, for example, containing different mixtures of chain lengths following alternative refinement procedures. With this discrepancy, there will be deviations in physicochemical properties of the materials, with consequent modifications in drug release and hence absorption. Additionally, several excipients used in ointments, and indeed in other topical formulations, may cause sensitisation or allergic reactions. Though rare, these can be severe and hence if a patch test indicates an allergic response to one of the excipients, then products containing the sensitising agent should be avoided. Ointments are usually prepared by fusion, heating the components to greater than the melting point of all the materials before cooling. Generally, the minimum amount of heating is advisable and constant stirring during cooling will provide a more homogeneous product; rapid cooling generally creates stiffer ointments than those prepared by slower cooling rates.

5.5.2.2 Creams

For pharmaceutical and medical uses, a cream can be defined as a semi-solid emulsion for application to the skin or mucous membranes. Creams are usually more acceptable to patients than ointments as they tend to be less greasy, are easy to apply, and can usually be simply washed from the skin surface. However, they tend to be less occlusive than, for example, hydrocarbon base ointments, and thus hydrate the stratum corneum less well, an obvious requirement for dry skin conditions.

An emulsion is a system of two liquid phases, one of which is dispersed as fine globules within the other. The globules can vary in size, typically from 0.25 to 20 μm in diameter, with emulsions containing predominantly large droplets termed coarse emulsions and those with a globule size around 5 μm diameter termed fine emulsions. Very fine globules with diameters down to 10 nm (i.e., little bigger than a micelle) can be prepared – these systems are termed microemulsions. The liquid droplets or globules form the disperse phase (or internal phase), whilst the liquid in which the globules are dispersed is termed the continuous phase (or external phase). If oil droplets are dispersed in water, then the system is described as an oil-in-water (o/w) emulsion, and conversely, if the disperse phase is water and the continuous phase is oily, then a water-in-oil (w/o) emulsion results. Typically, emulsions appear milky, except for microemulsions, which are generally transparent. Some microemulsions form spontaneously, but generally an emulsion is an unstable system which requires the addition of an emulsifying agent to improve stability. Without the emulsifier, the dispersed globules would collide, flocculate, coalesce to form ever-larger globules that would ultimately separate into the oil and water phases; this phenomenon is termed "cracking". The emulsifier reduces flocculation and coalescence by steric or electrostatic repulsion of the globules. Additionally, an emulsion can be stabilised to some extent by increasing viscosity of the continuous phase, thus reducing the mobility of the droplets and hence reducing the potential for globule collision. Many materials can act as emulsifying agents, including surfactants (anionic, cationic, or non-ionic), some proteins, polymeric hydrocarbons, or alcohols, and some finely divided powders such as bentonite.

Multiple emulsions can also be formed where, for example, water globules are dispersed within oil globules in a continuous water phase; such a system would be termed a water-in-oil-in-water (w/o/w) emulsion. An advantage of these systems is that a water-soluble therapeutic agent can essentially be dispersed in an oil droplet (within the water in an oil droplet).

Dermatological creams can be w/o emulsions, termed "oily creams" which tend to act as emollients and are used in cleansers. Since the continuous phase is oily, these creams are more occlusive than the o/w systems and can leave a protective oily layer on the skin surface as the water evaporates. More common are the o/w creams, or washable creams (also termed "vanishing creams") with a continuous aqueous phase containing oily globules. These aqueous creams are often rubbed into the skin where evaporation of the aqueous phase gives a cooling effect. Though clearly not depositing an oily layer onto the entire skin surface, o/w creams can deliver lipophilic materials to the skin, as well as water-soluble molecules from the continuous phase.

Describing drug delivery from a cream is difficult since the system is dynamic; the cream changes as the continuous phase evaporates and as the emulsion cracks. If a water-soluble permeant is applied in an o/w cream, then as the water evaporates from the tissue surface, the degree of permeant saturation in the water phase will rise. This could increase drug delivery markedly, especially if the oil phase inhibits drug crystallisation, allowing the formation of a supersaturated state, and hence permeation will be promoted. Conversely, if an aqueous permeant is incorporated into an oily w/o cream, then the oil can deposit on the skin surface, thus providing an additional barrier to permeation for the hydrophilic permeant. Further, as an emulsion cracks, the micelles formed from the emulsifier can trap the drug within the continuous phase.

5.5.2.3   Gels

Gels are typically formed from a liquid phase that has been thickened with other component(s). The liquid essentially forms a continuous phase with the thickening agent providing a porous scaffold to maintain the semi-solid consistency.

The liquid phase can be a polar solvent, such as water, an alcohol, or a non-polar solvent, and often solvents will be blended to provide the continuous phase. Numerous thickening agents are available, with the selection partly governed by the physicochemical properties of the permeant and by compatibility with the continuous phase. Simple gels can be prepared from water thickened with natural polymers, such as carrageenans or pectin, or by using refined or synthetic polymers, such as hydroxypropyl methylcellulose or Carbopol. A range of grades and molecular weight fractions of these polymers is available, but they are typically used at between 1 and 5% in the formulation.

In terms of drug delivery from gels, the continuous liquid phase allows free diffusion of molecules through the polymer scaffold, and hence release should be equivalent to that from a simple solution. Drug release from the polymer can be modified for very large molecules (macromolecules), for highly viscous gels and, in particular, for drugs that bind to the polymer in the gel.

5.5.3 SOLID FORMULATIONS

Solid formulations are seldom used to deliver materials to and through the stratum corneum since the powder must undergo a dissolution step prior to permeation. Without the co-application of a solvent, transepidermal water loss or skin exudates are generally unable to dissolve the applied powder. Topical sprays are available for depositing powders onto the skin surface, but these generally include a volatile solvent that dissolves some of the powder prior to evaporation (with consequent solute supersaturation and hence elevated drug delivery). Dusting powders are used to reduce friction between skin surfaces and antiseptic dusting powders are available.

5.6 TRANSDERMAL PATCH OPTIONS

5.6.1 TRANSDERMAL SYSTEMS

Transdermal systems have generally been divided into three generations. First-generation transdermal systems are responsible for the majority of products on the market to date. In this group, delivery is often limited by the barrier properties of the stratum corneum and relies on passive diffusion, such as from patches, metered sprays, or gels. There have been 20 or so drugs/drug combinations developed in this form over the last 30 years, with the majority being patches. Initially, these were in the form of drug in adhesive and/or reservoir systems and more recently in multi-layer matrix systems. Such developments in the technologies involved along with improved patient acceptability resulted in a surge in approvals in the mid-2000s. However, approval rates for new drugs in patches have slowed as the number of drugs with the required physicochemical properties, the required poor oral bioavailability, and the need for less frequent dosing and steady-state delivery lacking with the more conventional oral delivery has diminished.

Second-generation transdermal systems rely on permeability enhancement in some form, the most common approach being absorption enhancers. Some of the classes of excipient enhancers examined include Azones, pyrrolidones, fatty acids, alcohols, glycols, surfactants, and phospholipids (see Chapter 3). Amongst these, fatty acids, alcohols, glycols, and surfactants usually have a dual role as a solubiliser in addition to their potential enhancing capabilities. The choice and selection of such enhancers depends upon the formulation type and nature of the drug. However, consideration should also be given to the enhancers' potential pharmacological activity, toxicity, duration of action, enhancing mechanism (and reversibility), stability, and cosmetic acceptability. Alternative methods of enhancement include active systems such as iontophoresis which, along with increasing skin permeability by disrupting the stratum corneum lipids, should also provide an added driving force for drug absorption whilst avoiding deeper tissue injury. However, this has proved to be somewhat problematic with lack of success despite the investment spent on developing such systems (see Chapter 4).

Third-generation transdermal delivery systems involve techniques which have their effect on the stratum corneum alone. Such approaches produce greater disruption of the stratum corneum and thus more effective transdermal delivery, allowing the potential delivery of drugs without the normal limitations in physicochemical properties, including biological drugs such as proteins, peptides, sSiRNA, antisense oligonucleotides, and vaccines. The active techniques involved include iontophoresis (again), electroporation, ultrasound, microneedles, thermal ablation, microdermabrasion, and thermophoresis, and combinations thereof. Nevertheless, the issues of miniaturisation, patient compliance, and acceptability, safety and cost of goods, as with all the other generations, remains.

5.6.2 Transdermal Patches

A transdermal therapeutic system (TTS) or transdermal delivery system (TDS) is applied to the skin for the purpose of delivering a drug to the bloodstream, in contrast to a topical product, which is intended to deliver the drug *to* the skin rather than *through* the skin (Figure 5.5).

Initial commercial enthusiasm about patches was based on the success of few therapeutic agents in several simple patches that gained widespread approval from patients who liked a convenient sustained delivery system that was easily removable and which had therapeutic benefits. Thus, transdermal patches containing nicotine as an aid to smoking cessation and oestradiol for use in hormone replacement therapy were, and continue to be, highly successful. However, the early interest in delivering molecules from these systems was tempered by the limited number of molecules that could be delivered by this route. So, for example, the drug must possess the appropriate physicochemical properties to allow delivery across the skin, the molecule has to be potent enough to work at relatively low doses, and it must have a wide therapeutic window so that inter- and intra-patient variability in skin

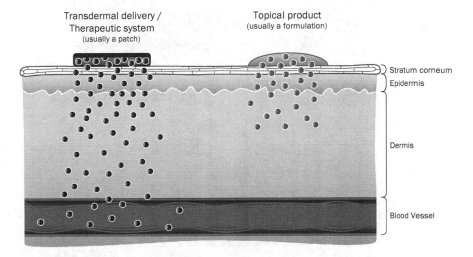

FIGURE 5.5 Transdermal vs. topical delivery.

permeability is problematic. Fortunately, scopolamine, nicotine, and oestradiol are ideal candidates for transdermal delivery; small molecules, appropriate lipophilicities and solubilities, and highly potent. There are few other molecules with similar properties – other oestrogens, androgens, glyceryl trinitrate, fentanyl, and clonidine – and these have also been successfully incorporated into patch devices. Attention then turned to examining the conditions where transdermal delivery could be useful. Thus, treatments for Parkinson's disease (parkinsonism), Alzheimer's, depression, ADHD, enuresis, and breakthrough pain have been developed. However, at present the markets are awash with "me-too" patches for delivering the same molecules, with the innovations arising from, for example, using a different combination of oestrogens, different patch components, or when a patch is used in combination with an active delivery approach.

5.6.2.1 Types of Transdermal Patches

The patches currently available can be categorised into three types depending on how the drug is incorporated into the device: those with the drug in the adhesive, those with the drug in a matrix, and those with the drug as a reservoir (Figure 5.6); the latter is becoming increasingly less popular as a result of adverse events associated

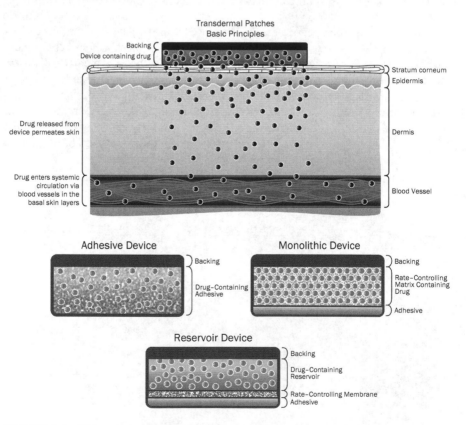

FIGURE 5.6 Three types of patches.

with product failure and subsequent dose dumping. Within these types, some variations are again evident, depending on the intended use of the patch. For example, the drug in adhesive type systems can contain one layer of the drug (for example *Nitro-Dur®*, Schering-Plough), or can be multi-layered where prolonged delivery is required, and each layer can contain increasing amounts of the drug to generate a concentration gradient within the system. Such a concentration gradient counteracts the increasing diffusion pathlength of the drug as the permeant depletes from the patch, thus maintaining near-constant delivery over extended times. This multi-layer approach is used for the delivery of glyceryl trinitrate from *Deponit®* (Schwarz) for the management of angina. Alternatively, the reservoir or matrix systems can have an entire adhesive layer or a peripheral adhesive for use where, for example, the entire adhesive layer would inhibit drug release from the device. Also, combinations of the above types have been generated where, for example, drug solids can be suspended in a solvent which is then mixed with a suitable cross-linking polymer to generate a matrix containing multiple micro-reservoirs of the drug.

5.6.2.2 Transdermal Patch Components

The European Medicines Agency (2014) describes the common features of transdermal patches as follows: "transdermal patches generally have an external backing layer which fixedly adheres the preparation containing the active substance(s). On the releasing side, the transdermal patches are covered with a protective film which is removed prior to application to the skin". The overarching description of patches therefore consists of (i) a backing layer; (ii) a preparation containing the active substance (which can vary in its composition); and (iii) a protective film or release liner. Several components in patch design are common between the patch types previously described. Thus, drug in adhesive, matrix, and reservoir devices generally all possess a release liner, an adhesive, and a backing layer. The reservoir devices (and possibly multiple drug in adhesive systems) utilise a semi-permeable membrane to regulate drug release. Beyond these components, the formulation of the drug reservoir is also important.

> **Release Liner:** The release liner covers the adhesive and is the layer removed
> to allow the patch to be stuck to the skin. These films can be prepared
> from polymers such as ethylene vinyl acetate, from coated papers, or from
> aluminium foil. Ideally, the release liner material must peel easily from the
> adhesive layer, without removing any of the adhesive, yet must be bonded
> firmly enough to the layer to prevent accidental removal. Thus, the release
> liner material is largely governed by the nature of the adhesive, with flu-
> orocarbon-coated polymer films used to line silicone adhesive systems,
> whereas silicone-coated films tend to be useful for systems incorporating
> acrylate-based adhesives. One further consideration in selecting a release
> liner is that it must be compatible with the formulation – usually being
> occlusive to minimise loss of volatile patch components (such as ethanol) –
> and that it should have good chemical stability.

> **Adhesive:** Clearly, the adhesive is a crucial component of all transdermal
> delivery patches, with devices generally utilising a pressure-sensitive

adhesive (PSA). There are generally three classes of PSAs used, though combinations of, for example, acrylate and silicone adhesives is common:

a. *Acrylate-based* adhesives are widely used in surgical tapes for holding catheters, for electrosurgical pads, etc. Acrylic adhesives are typically copolymers of alkyl acrylates, ranging from C_4 to C_8, with acetonitrile or acrylamide. Unlike some other PSAs, it is usually not necessary to incorporate other excipients, such as tackifiers or stabilisers into acrylic adhesives, and thus, as single component systems, they are generally less irritant than other PSAs (such as those based on silicone).

b. *Polyisobutylene (PIB)* adhesives combine different weight fractions of PIB with a liquid plasticiser, often a mineral oil. The various weight fractions of the polyisobutylenes have different properties; the higher molecular weight fractions give elasticity, whereas the lower molecular weight elements give tack. The polyisobutylene adhesives are highly flexible, but have less tack than the acrylate-based PSAs.

c. *Polysiloxane* adhesives are prepared by a condensation of linear polydimethylsiloxane gum with a silicate resin. The properties of the polysiloxane pressure-sensitive adhesives are thus dependent on the gum to resin ratio.

When attaching a transdermal patch to the skin, two stages occur during adhesion. Initially, when the device is first placed in position, the adhesive must wet the skin surface, so there is a liquid flow of the adhesive onto the skin. When the pressure is then removed from the patch, the adhesive must then fix. Thus, the pressure-sensitive adhesives above are viscoelastic, above their glass transition temperatures (T_g). Ideally, the PSAs should have glass transition temperatures well below that at which the device will be used (typically 32°C). With increasing difference between usage temperature and T_g, the initial adhesion of the PSA with the skin increases, but the fixation of the device decreases with T_g of the adhesive. Thus, there is a balance between the initial wetting stage and the longer-term fixation (or cohesion) of the device.

When selecting an appropriate adhesive, several factors must be considered. Amongst the desirable properties for the PSA are:

1. The adhesive must stick to the patient for the patch lifetime (may be up to a week).
2. The adhesive should be non-irritating and non-allergenic.
3. The adhesive should be compatible with the drug and other excipients.
4. The adhesive should allow the patch to be removed painlessly.
5. On removal, no adhesive should be left on the patient.

When used for extended times, patches can cause skin irritation. This is partly a result of the permeant, but also because patches tend to be occlusive with consequent hydration of the stratum corneum; whilst hydrating the stratum corneum is valuable for increasing drug delivery, it also poses some difficulties in the longer term. On extended use, the hydrated stratum corneum can encourage microbial growth, and the wet tissue can also adversely affect the adhesive performance. Both the polyisobutylene and polysiloxane adhesives have good water vapour permeability properties and hence reduce problems associated with long-term tissue occlusion. However, the polysiloxanes, whilst offering low toxicity and generally good skin compatibility, can themselves be irritating. One further problem, notable in drug in adhesive formulations, is that the drug can migrate through the adhesive layer on storage. This is usually not a problem with the acrylic-based polymers, but it is evident with polyisobutylene adhesives. Where this phenomenon has occurred, with delivery of scopolamine and clonidine, the migrated drug has formed an "adhesive depot" which provides a drug burst or pulse prior to pseudo steady-state delivery; the manufacturers have shown this to be a valuable method for overcoming initial drug:skin binding.

Testing skin adhesives is difficult. Clearly, the physicochemical properties of the system will be assessed (such as T_g) and this will give an indication of the adhesion properties: polyisobutylene adhesives have low T_g's and so provide flexible adhesives, but with less tack than the acrylate-based adhesives. Tack testing can be performed where the bond strength between a probe and the adhesive is measured after a short contact time under low pressure. Alternatively, the shear strength test is well-established (a British Pharmacopoeia method) for testing adhesive tapes, though it is not designed to mimic extended wear of transdermal delivery devices. Creep testing can measure the creep (or cold flow) of the adhesive and how the adhesive recovers on storage. However, wear tests are usually the favoured option when evaluating adhesives for transdermal delivery patches. These tests usually employ a placebo device (hence the properties may differ when an active permeant is incorporated), with volunteers using the device under different environmental conditions for the lifetime of the application.

Backing layer: The third common element found in the different transdermal patch configurations is a backing layer, and again, there are numerous materials that can be used in this regard. For example, the backing layer is usually occlusive when the patch is relatively small or when the active ingredient is surrounded by peripheral adhesive in the device, hence a polyethylene, polyester, or polyurethane backing may be selected. Some water vapour transmission is desirable for larger patches that are to be worn for extended times and hence less occlusive polyvinylchloride films can be used. Large patches also generally require a backing layer that has multi-directional stretch, as well as mechanical strength and hence a fabric-based backing layer may be valuable. It is essential that the backing layer is pliable to allow the device to conform to the skin (i.e., to move as the skin moves). Preventing cross-contamination is also an important function of the backing layer and particularly relevant for a compound such as rivastigmine, which affects neurotransmission and is associated with significant side effects.

Matrix: For devices incorporating the drug in a matrix, the composition of the matrix can dictate drug release. The matrices are often prepared using simple polymer mixtures, such as polyvinylpyrrolidone and polyvinylacetate with the drug dispersed or dissolved at elevated temperatures; the polymers then gel on cooling with the permeant incorporated. The relative proportions of the polymers modify the nature of the gel, and other excipients such as plasticisers (e.g., glycerol) can also be included in the matrix. Diffusion of the permeant through a polymer matrix is also controlled by the degree of polymer cross-linking and by the level of hydration in the gel. Hydrogels are alternative matrices formed from a network of hydrophilic polymers that are water swollen, but that are water insoluble.

Matrix-type systems will typically include a matrix layer containing the drug in equilibrium with its saturated solution to ensure maximum thermodynamic activity. To this an adhesive layer can be added which contains the dissolved drug in equilibrium with that of the matrix and which attaches the patch to the skin. Matrix-type systems can therefore be characterised as single-layer patches (where the drug is blended in the adhesive layer and there is no separate adhesive layer), or as multi-layered patches, such as "bilayer" patches (if an adhesive layer is added to the matrix itself; this is the case for Novartis' Exelon patches).

Semi-permeable (release) membrane: Transdermal patches were originally intended to control the delivery of therapeutic agents to the skin surface, with the implication that release from the device would control drug flux. However, the skin is such an effective barrier that it is the stratum corneum that is usually the rate-controlling membrane to transdermal and topical drug delivery. Thus, there may be little value in employing a semi-permeable membrane in terms of regulating drug delivery, but these membranes are used in reservoir transdermal patch designs, as well as in the multi-laminate drug in adhesive or matrix-type devices.

Many of the criteria described for other patch components also apply to the selection of the release membrane; it must be compatible, non-toxic, stable, et cetera. The membrane can be tailored to release the appropriate level of the permeant. Thus, a release membrane can be prepared from a copolymer of ethylene acetate with vinyl acetate. The proportion of vinyl acetate can affect the glass transition temperature of the film, with polyethylene itself providing a rigid glassy polymer with a low permeability, whereas polyethylene/vinyl acetate copolymers are more rubbery, with a greater permeability. Further, the release properties can also be modified (generally increasing membrane permeability) by the inclusion of plasticisers. Alternatively, microporous release membranes can be selected, such as cellulose ester films through which smaller linear molecules traverse more readily than larger branched permeants.

5.7 PREFORMULATION STUDIES

5.7.1 Overview

As defined in Section 5.4.2 ("Quality Target Product Profile"), there is a plethora of factors to consider when developing a topical or transdermal product. Nevertheless, preformulation in its truest form is a research and development stage where the drug's physicochemical properties and desired dosage form along with the drug's mechanism of action (drug target) and the disease are considered. For the development of topical semi-solid drug products or transdermal products, preformulation studies typically initially involve solubility and compatibility studies with potential excipients to be used in the final dosage form. Such studies are conducted to identify any critical parameters which may affect the development of the final product. These parameters may include poor drug solubility and achievable drug concentration, inherent drug instability, potential excipient/drug, excipient/excipient, device/drug (and combinations thereof) incompatibility amongst others. In addition, another aim of preformulation studies is to develop and explore methodologies to improve these defined issues such that the Quality Target Product Profile of the formulation dosage form can be achieved. Thus, preformulation studies are conducted to inform rational formulation design.

5.7.2 INITIAL CONSIDERATIONS OF THE DRUG

5.7.2.1 Drug Physicochemical Properties

The physicochemical properties of a drug that can influence its performance and manufacturability should be identified and considered during preformulation work and include, amongst others, log P (or log D), pKa, solubility and molecular weight. Such parameters play a key role in the inherent permeability of a drug across the skin as described in Chapter 3. The log P (log partition coefficient) reflects how well a drug partitions between lipid (oil) and water, whilst the pKa or dissociation constant is a measure of the strength of an acid or base and allows the determination of charge on a molecule at any given pH. Both measurements are useful parameters for use in understanding the solubility and diffusivity and/or partitioning across the stratum corneum. The selection and identification of potential drug salt forms or the use of a salt or free acid or base and a full understanding and characterisation of the solid state properties of the selected drug form is critical during preformulation studies, since these obviously influence drug solubility, stability, and ultimately, drug release and absorption. Such issues should be decided during the early development phase, since a change in form at a later stage may force repetition of toxicological, formulation, and stability studies, thus increasing development time and cost.

5.7.2.2 Drug Pharmacology (Target) and Efficacy

Given that the exact underlying cause of many skin or systemic diseases may not be well-defined or understood, the effective drug concentration required to reach the target site is also often not well-defined. Thus, before a decision is made to take a drug into topical or transdermal formulation development, several issues and questions should be considered (if they have not already been addressed in the candidate selection process):

1. Has the drug target or pharmacological activity of the drug been demonstrated or predicted, and what is the IC_{50} or minimum concentration required to exert a therapeutic effect?
2. What are the pharmacological models used in assessing and/or predicting the pharmacological activity of the drug, and are these models appropriate?
3. Is the target site known?
4. Is the drug metabolised?

For example, when targeting a drug to the epidermis, a highly potent drug with a low Kp may not necessarily be the most efficacious when compared to a less potent drug with a higher Kp, as it is a combination of a drug's potency and its ability to permeate the skin that is important. These parameters should be well-defined and understood during drug selection and during any preformulation work, since such information will allow proper evaluation of dosage form type, dose/drug concentration, and the selection of excipients.

5.7.3 PREFORMULATION

5.7.3.1 Solubility

Solubility plays an essential role as part of formulation development, since inadequate drug solubility in a formulation will impede drug development if the target dose cannot be achieved. Likewise, a very soluble drug may also pose issues such as poor drug release from a system. Thus, the solubility of a particular drug may necessitate the selection of narrow range of solvents which are only suitable for specific dosage forms. For example, a highly lipophilic drug is less likely to be formulated as an aqueous gel, but rather as a cream, ointment, or non-aqueous gel.

During preformulation study design, the selection of solvents is based on the initial dosage form of choice, using a library of topically acceptable excipients. Some of the approaches used to dissolve drugs for topical formulation development include the use of co-solvents, pH adjustment, complexation, surfactants, and a combination thereof. Of these approaches, the use of co-solvents is probably the most practical and commonly used method to solubilise poorly soluble compounds in aqueous systems. When sufficient solubility cannot be achieved in a single solvent (most likely aqueous), co-solvents are used as an alternative option to increase drug solubility. A variety of solvents can be used, and it is important that the selection of co-solvents is based on the miscibility of each solvent to avoid phase separation. In addition, solvents and non-solvents are also used in co-solvent systems to increase the thermodynamic activity of highly soluble drugs at the desired drug concentration. Altering pH is an effective method to increase drug solubility, since most drugs are weakly ionisable acids or bases and, with a consideration of the pH of the solution and the pKa value of the drug, solubility can be optimised. In addition, it should be emphasised that the pH of the final formulation should be in the region of 5 to 7, although slightly more acidic pH values may still be acceptable for topical formulations depending on the application site, dosage frequency, and area. Surfactant systems can also be evaluated, but recently, the use of emulsifier-free approaches has intensified in the development of pharmaceutical and cosmetic products. Creams or emulsion-based systems usually comprise one or more traditional emulsifiers such as surfactants to stabilise the formulation. However, due to the irritancy potential of traditional surfactants, polymeric emulsifiers such as carbomers, celluloses, and polyacrylates have been successfully used to stabilise emulsions and replace surfactants. The high molecular weight of such polymeric emulsifiers means that that they are less likely to penetrate the stratum corneum, thus minimising any of the unwanted effects often observed with surfactants. In addition, surfactants, like detergents and soaps, have a tendency to emulsify and remove natural lipids within the skin, leaving a "dry skin" feel, a drawback not observed with polymeric emulsifiers.

For the development of topical semi-solids, typically up to 20 solvents would be selected for solubility screening during an initial preformulation stage. The suitability and range of such solvents are initially selected based on the physicochemical properties of the drug and the desired dosage form or product profile to be developed. The completion of this initial investigation will determine if a wider range of alternative solvents have to be investigated or if the target dose can be achieved. If the latter is achievable, co-solvent systems would be developed, and together with the drug, these systems would be tested for drug/excipient and excipient/excipient compatibility.

5.7.3.2 Compatibility

Excipients are the components of a formulation that in combination produce a "successful" pharmaceutical product. Although the drug or active pharmaceutical ingredient is of primary importance since it is responsible for the treatment of the disease, in order to "present and deliver" the drug, excipients play an equally important role. Whilst, traditionally, excipients have been used as "inert" material, such as bulking agents in dosage forms such as tablets, more recent development of drug delivery systems has used the benefit of excipient–drug interaction to produce formulations with specific properties and performance specifications. Thus, any interaction between excipients and the drug substance must be well understood and is fundamental in developing any drug product.

Excipient/drug or excipient/excipient compatibility can be classified as physical, chemical, or physiological, and such interactions may have implications for drug stability, product manufacture, product adhesion, drug release, product efficacy, therapeutic activity, and side-effect profiles. There are several approaches to conducting excipient compatibility screening and, whilst dependent upon the dosage form, the main approach is based on accelerated temperature studies. In this case, an experiment is designed to investigate the effect on compatibility of the drug and excipient under real time (25°C) and accelerated conditions (40°C). Usually, such experiments are designed using excipients comprising solutions of the drug in pure solvent to investigate experimental "extremes". Higher accelerated temperature conditions may be investigated, but such experiments must be based on the assumption that any reaction rate is proportional to temperature, and this is often not the case. For example, based on an approximation of the Arrhenius equation (and assuming first order kinetics), a study performed at 40°C over a month would equate to a shelf-life of approximately four months at 25°C. Although the majority of initial excipient compatibility studies for topical dosage forms are performed on solvents and excipients existing as liquids at room temperature, consideration has to be taken of semi-solids with low melting points and the fact that in a patch the solvent would be dried off. For example, semi-solids such as fatty acids with low melting points employed as thickeners may have enhanced potential for interaction if the product is stored at elevated temperatures. Likewise, crystallisation of poorly soluble excipients at lower temperatures should also be investigated. Thus, the key objective of an excipient compatibility screen is to eliminate or mitigate any risks at an early product development stage for a particular drug or active substance.

For patches, compatibility of drug with the adhesive, other polymeric components of the matrix, or penetration enhancers can be performed in liquid or solid form but the issues of drug and/or excipient crystallisation/precipitation at different temperatures remains the same.

5.8 FORMULATION DEVELOPMENT

Although the specifics of a Target Product Profile for a formulation applied to the skin will vary depending on its ultimate purpose, there are key aspects of most target profiles that are the same for most formulations. The most basic of these is the use of approved excipients, where the type and concentration of excipient used should be acceptable from a regulatory perspective (as discussed earlier). It is also always the case that the excipients utilised must be suitable for use in the disease state for which the formulation is designed. The extent and rate of release of drug from a formulation should be well understood. *In vitro* release rates are a useful assessment of this parameter and can also serve as a valuable QC release tool in monitoring formulation changes on storage. Clearly, it should be demonstrated that the formulation should deliver the drug into the skin at the required concentration and to the required site of action or at the required systemic levels. The cosmetic elegance and patient acceptability of any dermal product is also important whilst the physical and chemical stability of the drug/formulation must yield adequate shelf-life. For patches, the wearability and adhesivity during product use is also critical, as is ensuring that the developed formulation can be manufactured at commercial scales. Lastly, the cost of goods for the product must satisfy the demands of its particular market. Ultimately, it is always important to remember a general rule that the simpler a formulation is, the fewer things there are to go wrong!

For chronic dermatological disorders such as eczema, psoriasis, and dermatitis, occlusive formulations such as ointments or anhydrous systems are often preferred since these preparations have protective properties. However, such anhydrous mixtures are also usually very tacky and greasy and have poor aesthetic properties. Although such formulation types are extremely useful as emollients due to their occlusive properties, their value as topical products is limited by the poor solubility of many drug substances in them. In such cases, drug solubility can only be enhanced by formulating them with hydrocarbon miscible solvents, such as isopropyl myristate or propylene glycol. Anhydrous systems may also comprise pure polyethylene glycol (PEG) systems or triglyceride derivatives in addition to the traditional hydrocarbon systems containing white soft paraffin and petrolatum. Alternatively, silicone-based formulations may also be used, however, the regulatory status of silicones for topical use is currently limited, even though an extensive positive safety profile is emerging.

Alternative monophasic systems to ointments are aqueous gel formulations. Such systems usually contain water-based or alcohol-based co-solvent systems with a thickening agent based on cellulose derivatives, polysaccharide polymers, or acrylate polymers. Although these systems are more aesthetically pleasing than anhydrous systems or ointments, they do not have the occlusive properties of the former systems and as such are usually used for the application of anti-inflammatories, anti-infectives, or anti-histamines, or where facial application is required, such as with acne and rosacea where occlusive properties are not required and such gels are less likely to leave a greasy "residue". To improve the occlusive properties of gels, "emulgels" have been developed. Emulgels, or emulsified gels, are essentially bi-phasic systems containing an aqueous gel dispersed with a lipid phase, closely relating to a cream.

As described in Section 5.5.2.2, creams are emulsion systems of oil-in-water (o/w) or water-in-oil dispersions (w/o). The indication for which the product will be used is an important consideration in the choice of emulsion type; o/w emulsions are significantly more commonly used than w/o, with a wider range of regulatory acceptable emulsifying agents available for stabilising w/o emulsions compared to o/w emulsions. In terms of cosmetic acceptability, o/w emulsions generally feel less "greasy" and thus more acceptable. The development of multiple emulsions, for example, an oil-in-water-in-oil (o/w/o) allows compartmentalisation of incompatible excipients/drugs with similar physicochemical properties in this multiple phase system.

5.9 SOME GENERAL FORMULATION RULES AND RISK MITIGATION

From the preceding chapters, it is evident that some general "rules of thumb" can be drawn for optimising the transdermal and topical formulation development process.

5.9.1 SELECT A GOOD DRUG CANDIDATE

In terms of passive drug delivery, the transdermal route tends to be appropriate for small molecules, with good lipophilicity yet a suitable aqueous solubility. Thus, molecular size should be limited to 300–500 Da, and the permeant should have a log partition coefficient (octanol/water) in the range 1–3.5. Transdermal drug delivery is generally restricted to relatively potent drugs, but which also have a reasonably wide therapeutic window, since there is considerable inter-patient variability in skin permeability. Typically, a "good" permeant will have a flux in the region of 1 mg/cm^2/day and hence from a realistic patch size of 10 cm^2 delivery will be in the order of 10 mg/day. Using the 1 mg/cm^2/hour estimate will generally give an indication of the maximum achievable dose for the therapeutic agent. When estimating doses, it is also important to bear in mind that first-pass hepatic metabolism is avoided, and hence a simple oral dose may not be that required by the transdermal route. Further, if local effects are required, then the oral dose can greatly overestimate the amounts that are required by the topical route.

Having fulfilled the above criteria regarding molecular size, partitioning, solubility, and daily dose, it may be expected that transdermal delivery of the permeant is feasible. Before progressing to formulation and *in vitro* studies, it is sensible to estimate drug flux through human skin. This can be done in several ways. The literature contains data quoting flux values for permeants traversing membranes. If a literature report uses a molecule with a similar structure (and hence similar physicochemical properties), then this can be a guide for the expected flux of the permeant under investigation. When using this analogous approach, literature data obtained on human skin are clearly preferable to those deduced from animal models or inert membranes, assuming that the experimental protocol is valid.

A second approach for drug candidate selection for dermal formulation development requires the use of mathematical models an attempt to predict dermal absorption *in silico*. Formulation scientists have been tempted, especially in the pharmaceutical arena, to find the most promising compounds by investigating the relationship between percutaneous permeation and molecular parameters such as lipophilicity (most commonly expressed as log P, the logarithm of the octanol–water partition coefficient), hydrogen bonding, molecular weight (or size), and melting point. Quantitative Structure Property-Activity Relationship (QSPR) studies have meant that, if a correlation is found, it is possible to screen any number of compounds, including those that have not been yet synthesised, for the selection of those structures with the required properties for the desired delivery. A range of non-linear methods have also been employed to improve predictions of skin absorption. Artificial neural networks (ANNs) have been investigated, showing high predictive power. However, ANNs are a limited method, in that they have a tendency to over-fit where large numbers of physicochemical descriptors exist compared to the data points used. Such models are often weighted and are susceptible to over-training. Gaussian process (GP) methods do not alleviate all these issues, but minimise them, reportedly providing better predictions of percutaneous absorption than existing models, perhaps suggesting that the approach of predicting skin absorption by means of a simple equation may have limited mechanistic value.

Despite limitations, there are a plethora of *in silico* models that exist for the formulation scientist to help identify the molecules that will be best absorbed. However, for the formulation scientist, other factors need to be considered – including predicted or experimentally derived molecule stability, solubility, irritancy, toxicity, and potency – before a final decision on candidate selection is made. Despite the developments in *in silico* modelling, they are yet to replace actual skin permeation testing using the type of *in vitro* models described in Chapter 6 and will probably remain as such until their reliability and correlation with experimentally derived data can be confirmed. As often is the case, it is experience rather than theory that guides the best way forward, and there will always be drugs that defy the rules.

For example, overcoming this size exclusion phenomenon could present a major disruptive breakthrough in dermal drug delivery. Tacrolimus and pimecrolimus (MW = 804 Da and MW = 810 Da, respectively) are the two most well-known compounds that seem to go against the molecular weight rule described above. However, the development of novel protein therapeutics or biologics has gained significant momentum in the biopharmaceutical sector in recent years with many of these actives subject to poor oral bioavailability due to their large molecular size and first-pass metabolism. Hence, despite the issue of molecular weight, successes of the passive delivery of amongst others, hyaluronic acid (ca. 500,000 Da) and an IL23 aptamer (ca. 30,000 Da) have been reported.

5.9.2 Selection of Excipients for the Formulation of Choice

5.9.2.1 Regulatory Perspective

Pharmaceutical dermal formulations rarely contain a single excipient, and vary markedly from systems with varying excipients from relatively few (e.g., aqueous gels or lotions; drug in adhesive patches) to greater than ten (e.g., emulsion systems). The simplest way to choose and utilise excipients is to select those with appropriate properties that are used in existing formulations that have received regulatory approval in the territories relevant to your product. The legislation and nature of regulatory control varies from one country to another; however, in general, acceptable pharmaceutical excipients are listed in international Pharmacopoeia with extensive published safety data. Notably, the use of existing excipients requires regulatory consideration when using an established excipient for an alternative delivery route. For example, the oral consumption of an excipient that has been used in a topical dosage form may well mean that additional toxicity studies are required. In contrast, an orally delivered and absorbed excipient may present fewer toxicological concerns (other than irritation) when applied topically as absorption will be significantly lower than from the oral route. Less extensive supporting data may be required if each excipient has extensive supportive toxicity data, previous approval for food use, has been used in oral administration or is already used cosmetically. However, although regulation of cosmetic topical formulations is controlled by legislation, these are generally less strict regarding excipient types, grades, and levels, and so a wider range of agents is available and acceptable than in the development of pharmaceutical topical formulations. As a consequence, it is clear that the general concept of "less is better" should be followed when developing a drug product. Thus, it is unsurprising that dosage forms with fewer components, such as gels, can often be favoured for development and manufacturing over the more traditional creams.

A transdermal patch, as with most transdermal delivery systems, is classified by the FDA as a combination product, consisting of a medical device combined with a drug or biological product that the device is designed to deliver. As such, the selection of acceptable liners and backing layers should also be taken into consideration in addition to excipients and adhesive itself in the case of a drug in adhesive patch. From a commercial perspective, the source and availability of any excipients or components used to develop the final product should also be chosen with care, since certain components may only be available from a limited supplier(s) which may in turn be exclusive to certain territories.

For any dosage form, the Inactive Ingredients Database (IID) provides a list of different formulation excipients already in approved products, along with the type of dosage form and the maximum level in a product approved to date. Generally, this is a valuable resource when considering development of a new topical or transdermal product.

5.9.2.2   Role of Excipients

Excipients typically comprise over 90% of a topical pharmaceutical product and are included to perform a variety of functional roles in such formulations. For the purpose of a semi-solid topical dosage form, such functional roles may include:

- Improvement of solubility to allow incorporation of the drug at the target concentration
- Controlling drug release and permeation
- Improving general aesthetics of the product to increase patient compliance.
- Improve drug skin permeability and/or deposition
- Improve drug and formulation stability
- Prevention of microbial growth and contamination

Additional functionalities for a transdermal patch include:

- Adherence
- Tack
- Cold flow
- Rheology/viscosity/creep/shear

For aqueous-based preparations such as aqueous gels and o/w emulsions, water is often the main drug solvent, although various water-miscible solvents such as polyols (e.g., polyethylene glycol and propylene glycol) and alcohols (e.g., ethanol, isopropyl alcohol, benzyl alcohol) can be included to improve drug solubility. Humectants such as glycerol, triacetin, and polyols have traditionally been included into aqueous-based formulations such as gels to improve the moisturising and occlusive effect gels lack in comparison to creams and ointments. Formulations with a high emollient content, such as lipids found in creams and ointments which, when applied to the skin, protect and soften the skin, making it more supple, are often used for dry and inflammatory skin conditions such as in patients with dermatitis, psoriasis, and eczema.

The stratum corneum provides a physical barrier to the skin from the external environment, and as a result, prohibits or reduces the permeation of topically applied drugs. In an attempt to reduce the barrier function of the stratum corneum, a vast range of chemical permeation enhancers has been evaluated with varying degrees of success. Some of the classes of enhancers examined include fatty acids, alcohols, glycols, surfactants, and phospholipids (described in detail in Chapter 3). Fatty acids, alcohols, glycols, and surfactants usually have a dual role as a solubiliser in addition to their potential enhancing capabilities. The choice and selection of enhancers depends upon the formulation type and nature of the drug; however, consideration should also be given to the enhancer's potential pharmacological activity, toxicity, duration of action, enhancing mechanism (and reversibility), stability, and cosmetic acceptability.

Antimicrobial preservatives are usually included in formulations containing water, such as aqueous gels and creams, to prevent contamination and growth of microorganisms. In non-aqueous systems such as ointments, it is uncommon to include antimicrobial preservatives, since microorganisms while they may survive, would rarely proliferate under such conditions. A preservative should be active against a wide spectrum of microorganisms, and its selection should be based on several factors such as compatibility with the formulation, toxicity, irritancy potential, and the site at which the formulation is to be applied. The concentration of preservative required should also be taken into consideration since the presence of other excipients within the formulation may have antimicrobial activity. Examples of some commonly used preservatives include alcohols (e.g., benzyl alcohol, ethanol, and phenoxyethanol), hydroxybenzoates (all salts), phenols (e.g., chlorocresol) and quartenary ammonium compounds (e.g., benzalkonium chloride and cetrimide).

5.9.3 PRODUCT "IN USE" CONSIDERATIONS

During product use, most formulations undergo considerable physical changes once they are applied to the surface of the skin. For example, the effect of rubbing may decrease the viscosity of a formulation containing a thixotropic gelling agent such as xanthan gum, and this in turn may affect drug release from the formulation and permeation across the skin. If a volatile solvent is present, evaporation of a drug solvent within a formulation may reduce the solubility of the drug and result in precipitation or physical instability of the formulation. However, this effect has also been used by many formulation scientists to increase the drug thermodynamic activity, and thus increase drug release. Oxidation reactions in products intended for multiple use may be accelerated because of potentially greater and longer exposure to oxygen after opening. In such cases, careful consideration must be given to the selection of an appropriate antioxidant and the conditions under which its efficacy is tested. Likewise, contamination from frequent use may warrant the inclusion of a preservative such that the microbial load throughout the product life remains below the recommended level. For patches, adhesion and cold flow are potential "in use" complications, but whatever the dosage form, drug stability, release, and permeability, along with dosage form stability and irritation all need to be considered.

5.9.4 THERMODYNAMIC ACTIVITY

As has been described earlier (Chapter 2, Section 2.5.2), the driving force for permeation is the thermodynamic activity of the permeant in the vehicle. Generally, maximum flux is obtained when the drug is saturated within the donor system, although enhancement of flux can be obtained by using supersaturation. Thus, when formulating for transdermal or topical delivery, the drug should be at its solubility limit. This simplistic guide does, however, present problems. For example, with a drug at saturation in its formulation at 25°C, when the preparation is applied to the skin with a surface temperature of around 32°C, the drug will no longer be saturated. More importantly, when the same formulation with the drug saturated at 25°C is placed in a cool environment, the solubility limit of the drug in the formulation will fall, the system will be supersaturated, and, as a metastable state, the drug will crystallise from the formulation. Further, the preparation of a saturated vehicle is relatively straightforward when using a simple one-phase donor such as water but becomes rather more difficult when more elegant formulations are employed. For example, when using emulsions, it is important to saturate the external phase, but partitioning of the permeant between the lipid/oil phase and the aqueous phase can present some difficulties in this regard.

As shown earlier, providing that the vehicle does not affect the barrier nature of the stratum corneum, then saturated solutions of a given drug should give the same drug flux, whilst solutions at various drug saturations will give different drug flux. Thus, when formulating topical and transdermal preparations, a relatively low concentration of drug can be incorporated by inclusion of an (inert) antisolvent in the formulation. However, there is a limit on how low the concentration of the drug in the formulation can be. For materials with low solubilities in the vehicle or with very high skin permeabilities, as the drug enters the skin, then the formulation can rapidly deplete of the permeant, and hence the thermodynamic activity of the system falls dramatically; a 10% depletion of donor concentration adversely affects delivery. This can be the case with, for example, steroids which, as lipophilic molecules, tend to traverse the stratum corneum well. To counteract depletion, a solid drug can be suspended in the formulation. The solid drug dissolves to replenish the donor phase and hence maintains the driving force for permeation. For this approach to succeed, it is necessary for the suspended particles to dissolve rapidly; again, this may be problematic when using highly lipophilic permeants (i.e., the materials most likely to suffer from depletion effects). Since the dissolution rate is dependent in part upon the particle size (from the Noyes–Whitney equation), then micro-crystalline drug particles are most likely to replenish the donor solution without introducing a dissolution rate-limiting barrier to permeation. However, the use of a suspension in dermal product development – although sometimes theoretically attractive – is often unfavourable in practice (see below).

5.9.5 BE REALISTIC WITH REGARD TO DRUG ENHANCEMENT AND LOCALISATION

Having selected a candidate with appropriate physicochemical properties, estimated a value for flux across human skin using some mathematical relationships and tested its flux across skin *in vitro* from a saturated solution, it is time for a "reality check". Again, it must be borne in mind that *in vitro* data only provides an estimate for *in vivo* delivery, but if the flux determined experimentally is grossly below that required clinically, then an alternative route of administration is indicated. Notwithstanding some of the newer technologies for circumventing the stratum corneum barrier, such as microneedles or laser ablation, "standard" formulations can at best improve flux through the skin by around an order of magnitude. Thus, if a component of a formulation such as a solvent, surfactant, or fragrance has some penetration-enhancing activity (e.g., ethanol, sodium lauryl sulphate, or a terpene), then drug flux could be promoted to some extent. Likewise, if a formulation contains a volatile element that is lost when the formulation is applied to the skin, then a transient supersaturated system will deliver the drug somewhat more efficiently than from the original formulation; again, around an order of magnitude increase in drug delivery is the most that can realistically be expected. Many oestradiol patches on the market actually deliver greater amounts of the steroid than would be expected from *in vitro* permeation experiments. This increased delivery is partly due to discrepancies in data from *in vitro* and *in vivo* studies, but also because some components may modify the stratum corneum structure, the patches are occlusive and so hydrate the skin thus enhancing drug flux, and some patch excipients are volatile (e.g., ethanol) and are lost from the device, thus supersaturating the drug in the system. In general, enhancers, supersaturation, and occlusion can improve delivery *in vivo*, but don't expect miracles!

Many topical preparations would ideally retain the therapeutic agent within the skin strata, with little or none of the agent traversing the tissue to enter the systemic circulation. Systemic side effects from oral therapies to treat, for example, psoriasis or acne can be severe, but topical treatments tend to minimise these as the dose required is generally reduced with local application. However, retaining the drug within the skin, and even within particular skin layers or at boundaries between skin layers (such as at the epidermal–dermal junction for psoralens in PUVA therapy for psoriasis) is still desirable for highly potent and toxic permeants. Such an ambition is even more difficult where the skin barrier is compromised, as with many diseased states.

One approach to localising delivery is to include a solvent within the formulation that rapidly permeates into the stratum corneum to form a "reservoir" – a modified solvent nature in the tissue into which drug partitions and is retained. Skin reservoirs are well-known for steroids where activity can be retained for many days, resulting from binding of the molecules to sites within the skin. However, localising and targeting drugs to specific skin layers or regions is at present beyond our capability, with only limited success in retaining therapeutic molecules within the skin and thus reducing systemic dosing. The general rule is that after entering the skin, a drug will keep on going.

5.9.6   ALCOHOL CAN HELP

Maintenance of saturation, as described in Chapter 2, is particularly desirable for longer-term delivery, such as from a transdermal patch. For shorter contact times (i.e., with finite dosing), then ideally a pulse of the therapeutic agent would be rapidly delivered to the skin. For improved finite dose delivery, an evaporating vehicle can be helpful. For example, alcoholic vehicles can improve delivery as described above – by modifying stratum corneum structures and by generating supersaturated states. In addition, alcohols tend to permeate the skin well, and hence can form a transient solvent reservoir within the tissue, thus promoting partitioning of a permeant into the stratum corneum. Clearly, clinical constraints may limit the use of an evaporating vehicle, since an alcoholic vehicle is not appropriate for application to an open lesion or dry skin.

5.9.7   USE AN APPROPRIATE ANALYTICAL METHOD

Most topical and transdermal formulations contain several or more excipients with potentially low levels of the drug; therefore, an existing analytical method available for a drug may not be suitable to detect and quantify the drug in the presence of the other constituents of the formulation. Thus, modification of such analytical methods is usually necessary. Ultimately the method will need to be "stability-indicting" such that it will be suitable for the resolution, identification, and quantification of drug impurities and related substances throughout the product shelf-life. Also, when testing the performance of a formulation using *in vitro* experiments such as the measurement of skin permeation, extremely low levels of the drug may need to be detected, necessitating sufficiently sensitive quantification of the drug. Such methods are often very different to those used for the identification and quantification of the drug and its impurities in the product. Whilst "fit for purpose" methods may be sufficient for the initial development stage, a fully validated method as outlined by the ICH guidelines (ICH Q2A, Q2[R1] and Q2B) must be implemented for the drug and its related impurities during characterisation and stability testing of the final lead formulations prior to clinical studies.

5.9.8   SOLUTION OR SUSPENSION

It is generally accepted that solid drug micro-particles are not topically absorbed and so the development of a suspension topical formulation is counterintuitive for the following reasons:

- Theoretically, the delivery of drug from a suspension would be sustained compared with that from a solution under infinite dosage conditions, due to constant replenishment of the dissolved drug fraction that permeates from the suspended solid particles. However, after topical application, the formulation is absorbed into the skin (and/or rubbed off), resulting in drug particles (from the insoluble fraction) remaining on the skin surface (unavailable to permeate).
- In addition, physical stability issues (i.e., agglomeration of particles) are common with suspension formulations. These effects are exacerbated with a higher undissolved particle fraction in the vehicle. Therefore, a preferred approach is typically to have a very low particulate content to maintain stability, which can limit replenishment of the dissolved drug that is then available for delivery across the skin.
- Typically, the development process of a topical suspension formulation is more challenging compared to that for solubilised formulations. This is due to the requirements of drug characterisation and stability, with both the soluble and particulate fractions, i.e., there are two dosage forms.
- The manufacture of suspension formulations is typically more labour-intensive, where extra care is required to suspend the drug within the vehicle (i.e., avoiding incorporation of excess air). Failure to do so can result in changes in the physical characteristics of the product (i.e., viscosity).
- Finally, the regulators will request evidence that delivery and efficacy is consistent throughout the shelf-life of formulations. This is particularly challenging in suspension formulations as drug solid state properties, uniformity, particle size, and soluble/insoluble fraction are likely to change over time.

Nevertheless, despite all the above, a suspension may warrant this expense and risk, as it is a dermal product form that is very hard to replicate and thus genericise.

5.9.9 DEVELOPING TO PROOF OF CONCEPT (PoC) OR A COMMERCIAL FORMULATION

It is often argued that a small company, typically funded by external investment, will always take their drug candidate into a formulation development program that is cheap and quick in order to develop a suboptimal/prototype formulation to evaluate the asset in a clinical PoC study, aiming to show efficacy to release the next tranche of investment or license it to large pharma. This will then require reformulation, and thus extensive bridging studies or even starting again, before a more realistic commercial product can proceed to full conventional clinical evaluation.

For large pharma, the converse may occur where the focus is on development risks and "killing" an asset based on an inability to meet the QTPP before any clinical evaluation. Once all criteria are met and "formulation lock" is achieved, then a full formulation development program is performed to produce an optimised, patient-friendly, and stable formulation with the intention that this will be the commercially viable and approvable formulation (formulation lock) taken into all phases of clinical evaluation. Obviously, again, the focus is to kill the asset if any criteria are not met.

There is no right or wrong answer to the best approach, and it often depends on the finance that is available for the development program, but listed below are some risks and issues associated with the above:

- The risk of producing a suboptimal/prototype formulation is that any failure due to safety, efficacy, or quality in the PoC study could have been addressed by developing an optimised "final" or "locked" formulation.
- If the PoC study with the suboptimal/prototype formulation is successful, it is far from guaranteed that a "final" formulation can be produced with the efficacy, safety, and quality required by the regulators whilst also satisfying the investors and meeting the acceptability required by the consumer/patient.
- A locked or final formulation may still require tinkering as things are learnt through the clinical program, and thus bridging studies may still be required.
- There are numerous topical products on the market, developed by small companies and licensed to large pharmaceutical companies, that would have been culled at a very early stage if they hadn't been taken into PoC studies before they were licensed.
- Having only one drug candidate focuses the mind to "how can we address this problem" rather than "that's a problem, drop it, we have other candidates".
- Lifecycle management is becoming increasingly important.

5.9.10 SYSTEMIC TOXICITY OF A TOPICALLY APPLIED DRUG

The risk of systemic exposure and thus the potential for systemic toxicity is often thought low for topicals (as described previously), because it is an application of a small amount of formulation 2–5 mg/cm^2 often containing less than 1% w/w drug to a relatively small surface area where permeation to a large plasma volume is low, but elimination is efficient. However, it cannot be ignored that some diseases cover a significant body surface area (e.g., psoriasis) where the skin barrier is damaged and the formulation applied contains a drug that is highly potent and toxic in a formulation optimised for delivery. As such, the risk of systemic toxicity needs to be evaluated early on with the appropriate studies.

5.10 FORMULATION OPTIMISATION AND SELECTION

The performance of a dermal formulation can be assessed using a range of methods depending on factors such as formulation type, target disease, aesthetic requirements (wearability and adhesivity for patches), and application site. However, four main parameters that form a key role as part of a formulation development program are the formulation stability, drug release, drug permeation, and target engagement/systemic levels. These are described in detail in Chapter 6, but it is important to remember that a formulation optimised for drug release and permeation is often more efficacious and may require a lower concentration of drug which may reduce the cost of the final product, drug irritation potential, and remaining pay load risk (for patches), and also maximise clinical efficacy.

5.10.1 FORMULATION OPTIMISATION

Formulation optimisation is a continuous process and several approaches can be used to optimise a product during the development stage; examples include using factorial design, single factor approach, and a systematic approach.

Factorial designs are commonly used during product development, particularly when different formulation components (e.g., excipient/excipient and/or drug/excipient) are thought to interact significantly. Since the identification of key contributing factors such as parameter type, level, and range is often difficult, the risk of potentially omitting a real parameter often exists. In addition, where key contributing factors cannot be identified, such designs could potentially lead to large number of repetitions for each variable in order to ascertain data validity, and interpretation of responses may not always be straightforward. As the name suggests, a single factor approach involves varying each factor in series and such an approach is normally restricted to single parameter responses and is mostly unsuitable for the development of topical formulations which typically contain multiple variable parameters. A systematic approach is more often used by experienced formulators, and in such an approach, key contributing factors are systematically determined. An example of such an approach is highlighted in the flowchart described in Figure 5.3 where the development process involves a series of preformulation tests prior to development and testing of formulation prototypes to identify lead candidates. Throughout this process, the prototype formulations developed are "optimised" according to the outcome from the series of experiments performed in relation to the aims set out. Under most circumstances, optimisation would usually involve larger changes during initial prototype development, whilst smaller changes would normally be performed following completion of *in vitro* testing of formulation prototypes, and it is at this stage where optimisation of a formulation is mostly referred to.

The completion of stability studies, *in vitro* release, and skin permeation studies, depending on the outcome, may result in the need for a significant change to the formulation and thus iterations of the performance tests described above. For example, drug recovery from the epidermal layer following a mass balance study, if found to be below the target concentration, may be a result of several factors:

1. *Poor or no drug release from the formulation.* Likely reasons for this may be drug binding to excipients, low drug thermodynamic activity, or drug crystallisation. Such a phenomenon would be obvious when an *in vitro* drug release experiment is performed.
2. *Poor inherent drug permeability.* The suitability of a drug candidate to permeate across the skin can usually be predicted by assessing its physicochemical properties. For example, hydrophilic drugs with an unfavourably high molecular weight (>600 Da) would be less likely to partition across the stratum corneum compared to a more lipophilic drug with low molecular weight. In some cases, the inclusion of penetration enhancers can remedy

poor drug physicochemical characteristics, but this approach is not a panacea for all such situations.

3. *Insufficient dose or drug concentration.* Such risks are usually mitigated by performing a dose ranging study to cover a sufficiently wide range of drug concentration. In some cases, alteration of drug concentration may result in significant re-development work.

4. *Drug metabolism.* Although the metabolism of a drug is less significant when using excised skin, some degree of metabolism, depending on the skin storage condition, may still be present and this parameter should be considered.

Such explanations could equally exist if adequate levels were not observed in the dermis/receiver fluid for a patch product.

5.10.2 Formulation Selection

Along with formulation stability, drug release, and skin permeation testing, other performance assessments can include: aesthetic and cosmetic acceptability (wearability) perhaps by a consumer panel, adhesion, tack, shear strength and creep resistance for patches using standard tests, and the use of preclinical disease models and early stage toxicity assessment if required. In addition, stability in various packaging materials may be determined. Ultimately, the objective is to test the performance of the developed candidate formulations in order to mitigate the risk of failure during clinical investigation. However, once all such assessments and formulation optimisation has been completed, one lead and preferably at least one back-up formulation should be selected for full characterisation and stability testing.

5.11 FORMULATION CHARACTERISATION AND ICH STABILITY

Detailed characterisation of a formulation is usually performed once the lead candidate(s) formulation has been defined. Formulation characterisation is performed to define a provisional product specification and methods of measurement for these parameters such that the capability or performance of a product can be monitored during ICH stability tests and to ensure that they remain within the set specifications throughout its shelf-life. For topical semi-solids, some examples of typical parameters determined are described in the subsequent text. Obviously for patches, these need to be adapted with adhesivity, peel, tack, shear, creep, and leak tests also being performed.

5.11.1 Formulation Characterisation

5.11.1.1 Macroscopic/Microscopic Appearance and Odour

Macroscopic or product visual appearance may include colour changes, absence of particulates and/or formulation appearance (e.g., phase separation of semi-solid formulations on storage) where such observations provide first-hand information on the stability of the drug product. Microscopic appearance to observe the formation of drug particulates could be determined using optical microscopy, or more sophisti-cated instruments such as x-ray diffraction. Development of odour over time could be a stability indication, for example, in formulations containing triglycerides which are prone to hydrolysis or microbial contamination.

5.11.1.2   Drug Content and Uniformity, Related Substances, and Degradation Products

A validated analytical method capable of measuring drug content and impurities at the required levels should have been established by this stage of the development program. Although the specifications for drug content of a topical product would typically range between 95–105% for semi-solids, the levels of impurities depend on the drug in question and thus will have to be justified and characterised according to the analytical method and drug product. Extensive guidance on the testing of drug products and related substances/impurities and new dosage forms is available in the form of ICH guidelines and from the EMEA (EMEA, 2006). The determination of formulation uniformity is especially important for bi-phasic systems such as emul-sions. For example, a lipophilic drug may be preferably distributed within the oil phase of an o/w emulsion; therefore, it is important to demonstrate that the drug is uniformly distributed within the formulation. Uniformity is usually determined by analysis of the drug content from sampling of the top, middle, and bottom of a bulk sample.

5.11.1.3   Preservative Content

For products containing preservatives, part of the product specification should be to ensure that the specified level of preservative is present. In addition, preservative effectiveness must be monitored as part of the final ongoing stability program, and this can be accomplished through analysis for the level of preservative previously shown to be effective and/or through preservative efficacy testing.

5.11.1.4   pH

The skin has a pH between 5 and 6.5 and, as discussed previously, the pH of a prod-uct can influence not only the solubility and stability of a drug in the formulation but may also affect its potential to cause skin irritation. Therefore, many topical products are formulated to be in that pH range. Although development of products with lower pH values (up to pH 3.5) may be necessary, such products would require considerable justification from a formulation development point of view, and such potentially irritable pH values may be acceptable depending on the product use and frequency as well as application site.

5.11.1.5   Rheology and Viscosity

Testing for rheological or flow properties of a drug product is normally performed for formulations with bioadhesive or mucoadhesive properties where the rheological property and residence time would have an impact on the performance or release of the drug product. Thus, for most semi-solids applied to the skin, viscosity is normally employed to monitor or assess the "thickness" of a product type. Changes in viscos-ity of a product can be indicative of changes in physical stability or performance of a product. For example, a loss in viscosity over time from a gel formulation could indicate a possible breakdown in the molecular weight of the polymer as a result of microbial contamination (common with polysaccharide-based polymers) and may therefore affect the overall physical stability of the formulation. Therefore, it is important that batches comprising of similar molecular weight range are used to ensure consistency between product batches.

5.11.1.6   Microbial Quality or Microbial Limit Test (MLT) and Preservative Efficacy Test (PET)

The inclusion of an MLT for a drug product is dependent upon the dosage form, and therefore typically used only for non-sterile products which contain sufficient water to support the growth of microorganisms. Therefore, semi-solid dosage forms such as ointments and other non-aqueous systems, such as non-aqueous gels with little or no water sufficient to support microorganism growth, would not be routinely tested unless an excipient or the drug within the product is susceptible to microbial contamination.

Most multi-dose products for topical application would contain a preservative or a combination of preservatives. A PET is performed, usually on aqueous-based semi-solids, to determine the minimum effective concentration of one or more preservatives required for adequate control of contamination. Thus, products are considered satisfactorily preserved if they meet the requirements set out by the Pharmacopoeia. The appropriate preservative system for a particular drug product should be demonstrated to be effective below its target concentration (typically between 70–95% of target concentration), where the antimicrobial efficacy of the preservative in the final product should be assessed during product development, particularly during stability studies and at the end of the proposed shelf-life using a test outlined by a Pharmacopoeia.

5.11.1.7   Sterility

Sterile semi-solid formulations to be applied to the skin are mostly for wound or burn indications, are single-use products, and generally comprised of topical gels or solutions. Since the method of sterilisation is dependent upon the formulation type, composition, and also packaging, such factors should be taken into consideration even during preformulation stage and sterility testing should be performed in the final packaging such that container closure integrity can also be assessed. It is also important that the relevant sterility test is performed according to territorial requirements, since the sterility test outlined within the USP has several significant differences from the EP, whilst the Japanese Pharmacopoeia (JP) tests are identical to that of the EP.

5.11.2   ICH Stability

Once characterised, the formulation(s) are placed on long-term accelerated and real-time stability studies performed at ICH conditions 25°C/60% relative humidity (RH), 30%/65% RH, and 40°C/75% RH (ICH Q1A[R2]). Such a study may span a period of at least two years and typical time points may include t = 0, 1, 3, 6, 9, 12, 18, and 24 months where all characterised parameters described in Section 5.6.1 are tested to monitor the performance of the product over its shelf-life. At the same time, the primary packaging materials may also be selected and investigated with the formulation as a final product.

5.12 CASE STUDIES

The following case studies are intended to illustrate some of the above principles and the approaches taken when developing topically applied formulations. Clearly the challenges faced, and their mitigation, will vary according to the nature of the drug, the disease or condition to be treated, and the need to meet both clinical and commercial requirements. Thus, the below are intended to illustrate the approaches and principles in developing, testing, and optimising formulations, rather than providing a detailed and generic formulation development programme.

CASE STUDY 5.1

AIM

To develop a topical formulation for the treatment of a monogenetic disorder of cornification.

TECHNICAL CHALLENGES

- Good cosmetic and emollient properties to manage the dry and cornified skin condition
- Three concentrations of drug were required 0.2, 0.1, and 0.05% w/w
- Drug is highly susceptible to oxidation and light

DEVELOPMENT APPROACH

Forced degradation experiments showed that the drug was highly susceptible to both oxidation and light, which included ambient laboratory light. To ensure the integrity of the data generated during the work was not impacted by the light sensitivity, control measures using not only amber glassware, but also amber light coverings were put in place.

Preformulation studies showed that the drug had poor solubility in a wide range of solvents, including water. However, good solubility was observed in a selection of water-miscible solvents, including PEGs, alcohols, and solubilisers such as Transcutol P. Unfortunately, preliminary drug/excipient stability experiments showed poor stability in all excipients. In parallel, the impact of including an antioxidant (butylated hydroxytoluene [BHT]) in key solvents was also assessed which showed no issues arose. As there are known synergisms between different antioxidants, a DoE screening study was performed to determine the optimum antioxidant combination prior to moving into the development of prototype formulations. Although the drug was poorly soluble in water, the good solubility in water-miscible polar solvents resulted in a number of possible formulation approaches, providing that an antioxidant system was included.

Since emollient properties of the formulation were highly desirable because of the dry skin condition, creams and PEG ointments were the preferred formulation types. The first approach developed an o/w emulsion and, given the poor water solubility, the saturated solubility of the drug in solvent systems with low levels of water was used – glycerol as a humectant and PEG as the main solvent were developed. Differing levels of other drug solvents such as Transcutol P and ethanol were included in an attempt to maximise drug loading. However, because o/w emulsions require a minimum level of water (between 25–35% w/w), only formulations on the lower end of the target concentration could be developed (0.05% w/w). The drug was soluble in PEG, and therefore a PEG ointment was investigated. This included a low molecular weight PEG fraction with a dispersed high molecular weight fraction to increase the viscosity of the formulation, and was a more suitable vehicle to incorporate higher levels of drug and so achieve the higher drug target concentration of 0.2% w/w. In order to mitigate the risk of chemical and physical instability, and to test the effects of various solubilisers on drug penetration/permeation, a range of PEG ointments were developed which included various solubilisers, such as propylene glycol and Transcutol P, along with the optimised antioxidant system.

CASE STUDY 5.2

AIM
To re-develop a topical PEG ointment formulation for the treatment of dry skin conditions.

TECHNICAL CHALLENGES
- The current PEG ointment formulation was showing signs of separation
- Good cosmetic and emollient properties to manage the dry skin condition should be maintained as in the original formulation
- A physically stable formulation is required while maintaining the product performance in terms of drug delivery
- Time constraints due to imminent preclinical and clinical studies

DEVELOPMENT APPROACH
Prior to formulation optimisation, methods to accelerate physical stability testing were developed and assessed using the original formulation as a control. These included centrifugation, freeze/thaw, and rheological assessment, and a combination of these methods were subsequently used to rank re-developed formulations. Lead formulations were principally measured using an analytical centrifuge approach that measures the extinction of transmitted light across the full length of the samples to more accurately predict long-term stability.

The original PEG ointment formulation contained low levels of ethanol, water, and a penetration enhancer (Arlasolve DMI), in combination with high and low molecular weight PEGs. As such, a preliminary round of formulations was prepared and assessed for physical stability issues using the above methods, where each excipient was removed individually from the original formulation to ascertain if there was a single excipient which played a role in the physical instability issues (separation) that had been reported. The data generated was inconclusive, since physical stability issues were observed in all the formulations where ethanol, water, and the penetration enhancer had been individually removed.

In view of the time constraints due to the imminent pivotal preclinical and clinical studies, the decision was made to proceed with a less empirical, iterative stepwise approach where typically a single factor is changed at a time and is used to inform the next step and use a DoE approach. In this case, the input factors were the inclusion of non-PEG excipients and the ratio of high molecular weight to low molecular weight PEG and the output factors were the physical stability of the ointment. The output from the DoE indicated that while the inclusion of non-PEG excipients did have a detrimental effect on ointment physical stability (depending on level), it was the ratio of low to high molecular weight PEG that exhibited the most marked effect. The data was used to plot a design space, and a range of optimal mixtures within the design space – including different penetration enhancers – were selected for comparison of skin permeation/penetration to the original formulation. The performance testing data resulted in formulations that were similar in terms of skin permeation/penetration to the original formulation, and therefore a lead formulation was selected which contained the same excipients but at different levels to the original formulation.

CASE STUDY 5.3

AIM

To identify the lead compound and develop a topical formulation for the treatment of psoriasis.

TECHNICAL CHALLENGES

- Drugs had poor water solubility
- Drugs were highly susceptible to heat ($\geq 40°C$), and acidic ($<pH\ 4$) and basic ($>pH\ 9$) environments

PROOF OF CONCEPT

Prior to a full formulation development program, a "proof of concept" study was performed to determine if either (of two) drugs were suitable candidates for topical delivery. Initially, preformulation work showed both drugs were more chemically stable in oils such as castor oil, isopropyl myristate, liquid paraffin, and octyldodecanol compared to water and water-miscible excipients such as polyethylene glycols and diethylene glycol monoethyl ether. The drugs were prepared in oil-based solvent systems for permeation/penetration experiments to compare drug permeability.

The human skin permeation/penetration investigation showed compound 1 to be in the tissue at levels greater than the EC_{50} (albeit only 5000-fold higher), and at much higher levels than compound 2.

Based on the preformulation data, oleaginous ointments were identified as the most promising formulation type to maintain drug chemical stability. The use of white soft paraffin and stearic acid in combination with oil-based solvent systems provided initial oleaginous ointment formulations with desirable aesthetics (spread, texture, viscosity) with a target drug loading of between 1 and 2% w/w. As the manufacturing process for ointments included melting of the solid phase, the process was screened to ensure that the drug remained chemically stable when heated to 65°C in the solvent system, mixed in with the melted solid phase and then cooled to ambient temperature over various lengths of time. While the drug remained chemically stable throughout the manufacture process, it became apparent that there were incompatibility issues of the drug with some of the excipients following short-term stability screening. After a storage period of two weeks at 25°C and 40°C, the drug degraded by 10 and 30%, respectively. Alternative solid phase excipients were used in combination with the oil-based solvent systems to produce various oleaginous ointments, such as glyceryl monostearate, lanolins, hard fats, cetostearyl alcohol, and cetomacrogols. These changes resulted in improved drug stability, and were best in systems with only white soft paraffin, glyceryl monostearate, and/or hard fats.

Variations of these formulations were manufactured with and without different potential skin penetration enhancers in the oil-based solvent systems, such as isopropyl myristate and oleyl alcohol, and the human skin permeation/penetration investigations were repeated. The formulation optimisation and modification showed even greater levels of the drug could be delivered to the skin and illustrates that when formulation development is well-performed, then drug delivery can be optimised.

BIBLIOGRAPHY

Abraham, M.H., Martins, F., and Mitchell, R.C. (1997). Algorithms for skin permeability using hydrogen bond descriptors: the problem of steroids. *J. Pharm. Pharmacol.* 49: 858–865.

Barratt, M.D. (1995). Quantitative structure activity relationships for skin permeability. *Toxicol. In Vitro* 9: 27–37.

Barry, B.W. and Woodford, R. (1982). Optimisation of bioavailability of topical steroids: thermodynamic control. *J. Invest. Dermatol.* 79: 388–391.

Brown, M.B. (2005). The lost science of formulation. *Drug Deliv. Technol.* 10: 1405–1407.

Brown, M.B. (2008). The next generation in topical drug delivery. *Drug Deliv. Rep.* winter 24–26.

Brown, M.B. and Lim, S.T. (2012). Topical product development. In: Benson, H. and Watkinson, A.C. (Eds.), *Transdermal and Topical Drug Delivery: Principles and Practice*. New Jersey: Wiley, pp. 255–286.

Cronin, M.T.D., Dearden, J.C., Moss, G.P., and Murray-Dickson, G. (1999). Investigation of the mechanism of flux across human skin in vitro by quantitative structure-permeability relationships. *Eur. J. Pharm. Pharmacol.* 7: 325–330.

Degim, I.T., Hadgraft, J., Ilbasmis, S., and Ozkan, Y. (2003). Prediction of skin penetration using artificial neural network (ANN) modelling. *J. Pharm. Sci.* 92: 656–664.

EMEA (2006). *ICH Topic Q 3 B (R2) Impurities in New Drug Products*. CPMP/ICH/2738/99. London, UK: EMEA.

EMA (2014) Guideline on quality of transdermal patches EMA/CHMP/QWP/608924/2014

Farahmand, F. and Maibach, H.I. (2009). Estimating skin permeability from physicochemical characteristics of drugs: a comparison between conventional models and an in vivo based approach. *Int. J. Pharm.* 375: 41–47.

Flynn, G.L. (1990). Physicochemical determinants of skin absorption. In: Gerrity, T.R. and Henry, C.J. (Eds.), *Principles of Route-to-Route Extrapolation for Risk Assessment*. New York, NY: Elsevier, pp. 93–127.

Food and Drug Administration (FDA) (2004). *Guidance for Industry: PAT – A Framework for Innovative Pharmaceutical Development, Manufacturing, and Quality Assurance*. Rockville, MD: U.S. Department of Health and Human Services.

Food and Drug Administration Center for Drug Evaluation and Research (CDER) (2016). *Manual of Policies and Procedures MAPP 5016.1. Applying ICH Q8(R2), Q9, and Q10 Principles to CMC Review*. [Online] Available at: www.fda.gov [Accessed November 27, 2016].

Fowler, M. (2015). *Quality by Design (QbD) Approach to Generic Transdermal or Topical Product Development*. [Online] Available at: http://www.americanpharmaceuticalreview.com/Featured-Articles/172883-Quality-by-Design-QbD-Approach-to-Generic-Transdermal-or-Topical-Product-Development/ [Accessed February 18, 2016].

Food and Drug Administration (FDA) (1997). *Guidance for Industry. Nonsterile semisolid dosage forms. Scale-up and Postapproval Changes: Chemistry, Manufacturing, and Controls; In Vitro Release Testing and In Vivo Bioequivalence Documentation*, FDA, CDER, May 1997, SUPAC-SS, CMC 7. Rockville, MD: U.S. Department of Health and Human Services.

ICH (1995). Q2A: Text on validation of analytical procedures: Definitions and terminology. *ICH Harmonised Tripartite Guideline.*

ICH (1996a). Q2B: Validation of analytical procedures: Methodology. *ICH Harmonised Tripartite Guideline.*

ICH (1996b). Q2(R1): Validation of analytical procedures: Methodology. *ICH Harmonised Tripartite Guideline.*

ICH (2003). Q1A(R2): Stability testing of new drug substances and products. *ICH Harmonised Tripartite Guideline.*

ICH (2009). Q8(R2): Pharmaceutical development. *ICH Harmonised Tripartite Guideline.*

ICH (2005). Q9: Quality risk management. *ICH Harmonised Tripartite Guideline.*

ICH (2008). Q10: Pharmaceutical quality systems. *ICH Harmonised Tripartite Guideline.*

ICH (2009). Q8 (R2): Pharmaceutical development. *ICH Harmonised Tripartite Guideline.*

ICH (2010). Implementation of ICH Q8, Q9, Q10. *ICH Harmonised Tripartite Guideline*

Kirchner, L.A., Moody, R.P., Doyle, E., Bose, R., Jeffery, J., and Chu, I. (1997). The prediction of skin permeability by using physicochemical data. *ATLA Altern. Lab. Anim.* 25: 359–370.

Lionberger, R., Lee, S., Raw, A., and Yu, L. (2008). Quality by design: concepts for ANDAs. *AAPS J.* 10(2): 268–276.

Moss, G.P. and Cronin, M.T.D. (2002). Quantitative structure-permeability relationships (QSPRs) for percutaneous absorption: re-analysis of steroid data. *Int. J. Pharm.* 238: 105–109.

Moss, G.P., Sun, Y., Prapopoulou, M., Davey, N., Adams, R., Pugh, W.J., and Brown, M.B. (2009). The application of Gaussian processes in the prediction of percutaneous absorption. *J. Pharm. Pharm.* 61: 1147–1153.

Neumann, D., Kohlbacher, O., Merkwirth, C., and Lengauer, T. (2006). A fully computational model for predicting percutaneous drug absorption. *J. Chem. Inf. Model.* 46: 424–429.

Potts, R.O. and Guy, R.H. (1992). Predicting skin permeability. *Pharm. Res.* 12: 663–669.

Pugh, W.J. and Hadgraft, J. (1994). An initial prediction of human skin permeability coefficients. *Int. J. Pharm.* 103: 163–178.

Pugh, W.J., Roberts, M., and Hadgraft, J. (1996). Epidermal permeability – penetrant structure relationships: 3. The effect of hydrogen bonding interactions and molecular size on diffusion across the stratum corneum. *Int. J. Pharm.* 138: 149–165.

Rasmussen, C.E. and Williams, C.K.I. (2006). *Gaussian Processes for Machine Learning*. Cambridge, MA: The MIT Press.

Smith, E.W., Surber, C., and Maibach, H.I. (1999). Topical dermatological vehicles: a holistic approach. In: Bronaugh, R.L. and Maibach, H.I. (Eds.), *Percutaneous Absorption; Drugs – Cosmetics – Mechanisms – Methodology*, 3rd edn. New York, NY: Marcel Dekker Inc, Chapter 45, pp. 779–788.

Valenta, C. and Hadgraft, J. (2000). pH, pKa and dermal delivery. *Int. J. Pharm.* 200: 243–247.

Walters, K.A., and Brain, K.R. (2002). Dermatological formulation and transdermal systems. In: Walters, K.A. (Ed.), *Dermatological and Transdermal Formulations*. New York, NY: Marcel Dekker Inc, Chapter 7, pp. 319–399.

Williams, A.C. and Barry, B.W. (2004). Penetration enhancers. *Adv. Drug Deliv.* 56: 603–618.

Wilschut, A., Tenberge, W.F., and Robinson, P.J. (1995). Estimating skin permeation – the validation of 5 mathematical skin permeation models. *Chemosphere* 30 (7): 1275–1296.

Yamashita, Y. and Hashida, M. (2003). Mechaniostic and empirical modelling of skin permeation of drugs. *Adv. Drug Deliv. Rev.* 55: 1185–1199.

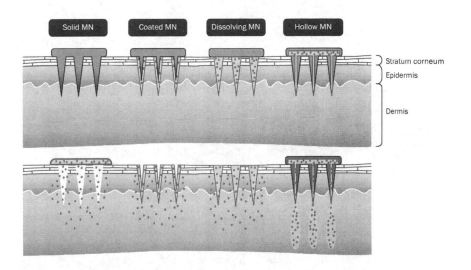

FIGURE 4.1 Illustration of the principal types of microneedles available and their typical dosing sites.

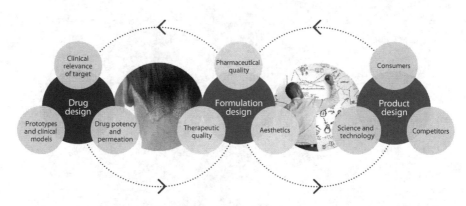

FIGURE 5.1 Common considerations for topical product development.

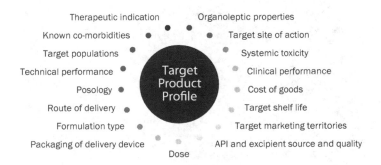

FIGURE 5.2   Considerations for a Target Product Profile.

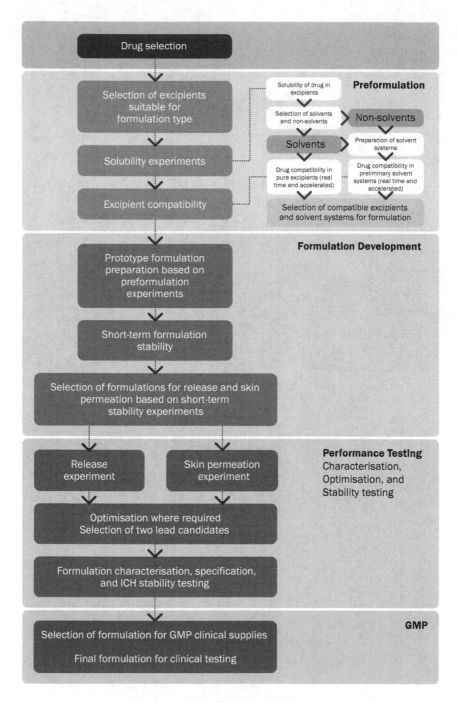

FIGURE 5.3 Flowchart summarising key events of a typical topical semi-solid formulation development program.

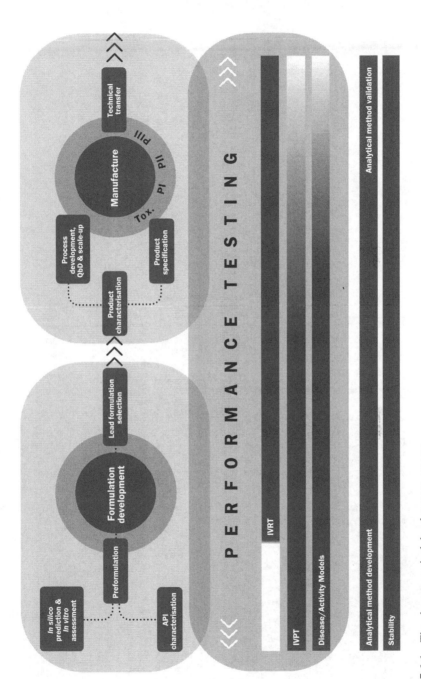

FIGURE 6.1 The pharmaceutical development process.

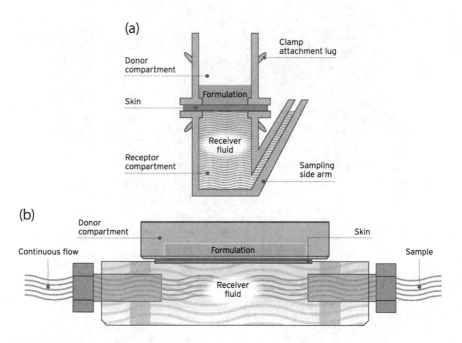

FIGURE 6.2 Schematic examples of (a) a static (Franz type) diffusion cell and (b) a flow-through (MedFlux) diffusion cell.

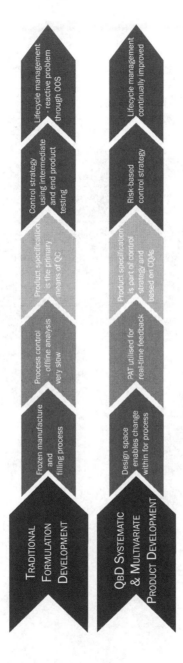

FIGURE 7.5 Comparing traditional pharmaceutical formulation development with a QbD approach. (From ICH, 2009. Q8[R2]: Pharmaceutical development. *ICH Harmonised Tripartite Guideline.*)

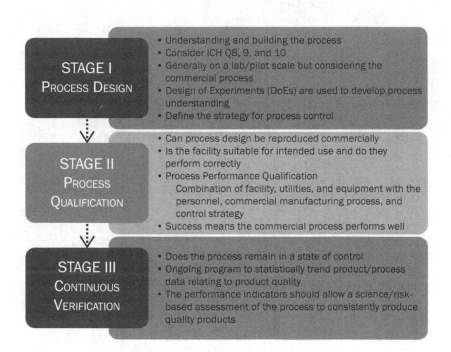

FIGURE 7.6 An overview of the process validation lifecycle approach.

6 Performance Testing

6.1 INTRODUCTION

Performance testing is an integral part of any formulation development program and can be used strategically throughout the development process to mitigate development risks and failures due to inadequate product performance. It is obvious that topical and transdermal formulations are for the treatment of patients *in situ*, and so the "gold standard" in the experimental design for formulation development would be to employ human volunteers and monitor drug delivery *in vivo*. In practical terms, this is extremely difficult for most drugs (e.g., New Chemical Entities – NCEs, and New Molecular Entities – NMEs), and would be unethical and cost prohibitive for formulation development or for studies on mechanisms by which drug delivery can be enhanced. Performing pharmacokinetic studies in humans for transdermal formulations where the intent is to deliver the drug systemically with drugs of known safety is well-established. In addition, for topical steroid formulations, *in vivo* studies have been performed, typically using vasoactive agents with measurements of pharmacological activity such as blanching used to assess drug delivery. Such vasoconstrictor studies have been useful for researching dose dependencies, or the influence of thermodynamic activity on drug delivery, but are necessarily limited and do not transpose to allow predictions for delivery of other therapeutic agents. Other *in vivo* techniques that have been used including skin stripping using adhesive tapes or cyanoacrylate glue, the use of punch biopsies, suction blister techniques, various forms of microdialysis, and non-invasive determinations such as confocal laser scanning microscopy, confocal Raman spectroscopy, or attenuated total reflectance Fourier transform infrared (ATR-FTIR) all have their merits. Animals are a potential alternative, but it has long been established that, other than toxicological studies (with many arguing this too is not appropriate), these have questionable relevance.

For transdermal patches, a variety of techniques exist which test both product quality and performance. Three types of adhesive tests are generally performed: the peel adhesion test, the tack test, and the shear strength test. The peel adhesion test measures the force required to peel away a transdermal patch attached to a stainless steel test panel substrate. The tack test is used to measure the tack adhesive properties where a test probe touches the adhesive surface with light pressure, and the force required to break the adhesion after a brief period of contact is measured. The shear strength or creep compliance test is a measure of the cohesive strength of the patch. Two types of shear testing are performed: dynamic and static. During dynamic testing, the patch is pulled from the test panel at a constant rate. With the static test, the patch is subjected to a shearing force by means of a suspended weight. Other tests involve evaluation of leakage to determine sudden drug release, creep resistance to measure cold flow (adhesive migration), and various other rheological techniques to assess the viscoelastic properties of the adhesive.

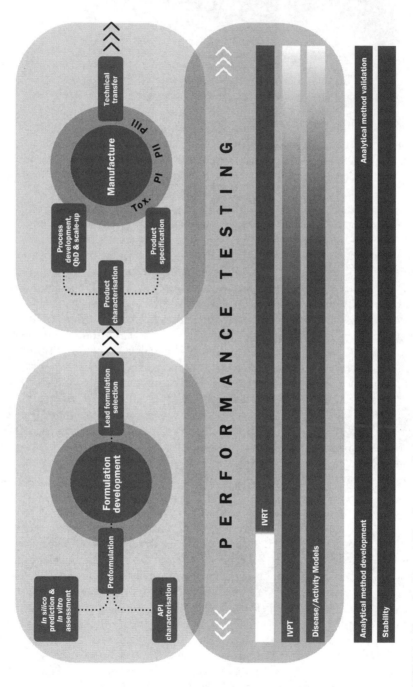

FIGURE 6.1   (See color insert.) The pharmaceutical development process.

Nevertheless, for both topical and transdermal products, the ability to measure drug release and activity from the dosage form in a reproducible and reliable manner is extremely important. In addition, any method should be capable of detecting changes in drug release/activity characteristics as a result of changes in active or inactive/inert ingredients in the formulation, physical or chemical attributes of the finished preparation, manufacturing variables, shipping and storage, age, and other critical quality characteristics of the finished product. When based on sound scientific principles, product performance tests can be used for pre- and post-manufacturing purposes such as during the product research and development phase, as a basic quality control tool, for demonstrating product similarity, or for demonstrating compliance with regulatory guidelines. Thus, for the remainder of this chapter: *in vitro* (drug) release testing (IVRT); *in vitro* (*ex vivo*) drug permeation and penetration (IVPT), and activity/disease models (DM) will be the focus.

Where these tests usually fit within a development process is schematically represented in Figure 6.1. However, some investigations are designed to answer specific questions, and so experimental methodologies may be specifically designed to answer these questions. Nevertheless, when designing experimental protocols for use in topical/transdermal drug delivery research, there are some guiding principles that should be followed. Inappropriate experimental design can provide misleading data that at best can confuse, and at worst can be dangerous if translated to a clinical situation. Thus, regulatory and advisory bodies produce guidelines and recommendations for methods to use when evaluating topical and transdermal drug delivery, and the current guidance/recommendations for IVRT, IVPT, and the use of skin disease models is detailed herein.

6.2 *IN VITRO* DRUG RELEASE TESTING

Absorption of drugs into (topical) and across skin into the blood supply (transdermal) depends upon a number of factors, including composition of the vehicle, type and condition of the skin barrier, and external factors (temperature, humidity, and occlusion). The factor with perhaps the greatest influence on the rate or extent of percutaneous absorption is the thermodynamic activity of the drug, which is influenced by its physicochemical properties such as solubility, molecular size, log P and ionisation state, and ultimately by its solubility in the solvents in which it is formulated. Drug release/dissolution methods for transdermal patches include U.S. Pharmacopeia (USP) Apparatus 5 (Paddle over Disk Method), Apparatus 6 (Rotating Cylinder Method), and Apparatus 7 (Reciprocating Holder Method). However, the method that is commonly used for both topical and transdermal dosage forms is that of *in vitro* (drug) release testing.

Synthetic membranes have been investigated extensively as a readily available and easy-to-use tool to study the *in vitro* release profiles of drugs from topical formulations to assess and compare product performance and quality. Examples of artificial membranes used include PTFE, polycarbonate, cellulose, and combinations of these. Such membranes can provide additional information contributing to the understanding of mechanistic aspects of drug delivery. For example, the thermodynamic effects of drug particle size and dissolution, drug solubility, partition coefficient, and pH and drug-excipient interactions can sometimes be better understood by using synthetic membranes. When a formulation is applied to the skin, the drug must first diffuse across the formulation, and the thermodynamic activity must then be sufficient for the drug to be released and partition into the stratum corneum. As such, this method is routinely used to optimise formulations for drug release prior to interface with the stratum corneum. In addition, like classical tablet dissolution testing, *in vitro* release testing has also been employed to demonstrate "sameness" under certain scale-up and post-approval changes for semi-solid products (CDER, 1997), and it is assumed that *in vitro* release testing can be used to characterise performance characteristics of a finished topical dosage form (i.e., semi-solids such as creams, gels, and ointments). Important changes in the characteristics of a drug product formula or the thermodynamic properties of the drug(s) should lead to a difference in drug release. In addition, methods of IVRT with significantly greater levels of validation are increasingly being used as routine quality control tools for product performance throughout QbD, process development, and scale-up, and for shelf-life studies. Also, over recent years, the U.S. Food and Drug Administration (FDA) have produced numerous draft guidance documents which include greater detail on validation of IVRT as a method, in combination with *in vitro* and *in vivo* bioequivalence studies, to show equivalence between a branded product and a generic (Q1–Q3) copy without the need for clinical studies.

6.2.1 IVRT METHOD DESIGN

A typical IVRT method for topical and transdermal dosage forms is most commonly based on an open chamber vertical diffusion cell (VDC) system such as a Franz cell system, usually fitted with a synthetic membrane (Figure 6.2). However, many other cell designs exist as specified in USP 40 General Information <1724> and can be used with suitable validation.

In general terms, the test product is placed on the upper side of the membrane as an infinite dose in the open donor chamber of the diffusion cell and a receptor fluid is placed on the other side of the membrane in a receptor cell. Diffusion of the drug from the topical product across the membrane is monitored by assay of sequentially collected samples from the receptor fluid. Aliquots removed from the receptor phase can be analysed for drug content by high-pressure liquid chromatography (HPLC) or other analytical methodology as appropriate (for example, mass spectrometry [MS]). A plot of the amount of the drug released per unit area ($\mu g/cm^2$) against the square root of time yields a straight line (when at steady state), the slope of which is representative of the release rate. Some methodological details required by regulatory authorities for IVRT include:

Method Parameters: Information should be provided to support the selection of the IVRT apparatus, product dose amount and application, sampling times, stirring/agitation rate, and any other parameters of the test method.

Membrane selection: Information on drug membrane binding and chemical compatibility with relevant receptor solutions should be provided to confirm the inertness of the membrane selected, and information on the linearity and precision of the resulting drug release rate in an IVRT should be provided to support the selection of a non-rate limiting membrane for the test method.

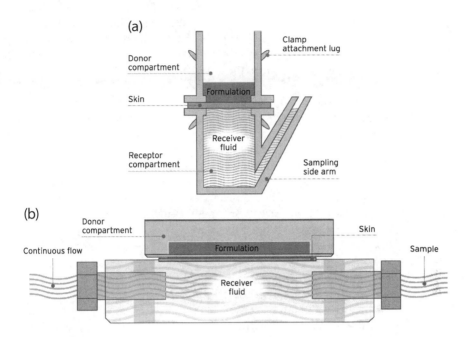

FIGURE 6.2 **(See color insert.)** Schematic examples of (a) a static (Franz type) diffusion cell and (b) a flow-through (MedFlux) diffusion cell.

Receptor Solution: Information on the empirical solubility and stability of the drug in the receptor solution should be provided to ensure that the drug is stable and does not exceed sink conditions throughout the study duration. In addition, information on the linearity and precision of the resulting drug release rate in an IVRT should be provided to support the selection of a receptor solution for the test method.

IVRT Method Validation: The apparatus, methodologies, and study conditions utilised in the IVRT pivotal study should be appropriately validated, qualified, verified, and/or justified. Detailed protocols and well-controlled study procedures are recommended to ensure precise control of dosing, sampling, and other IVRT study variables or potential sources of experimental bias. The validation of the IVRT method should incorporate the following qualifications and controls, performed using validated sample analytical procedures, as applicable:

IVRT Apparatus Qualification: Suitable apparatus examples for the IVRT method are described in USP 40 <1724>. The laboratory qualification of each diffusion cell should, at a minimum, qualify the diffusional area of the orifice in which the membrane is mounted, the volume of the receptor solution compartment in each diffusion cell, the control of a 32°C ± 1°C temperature (at the membrane), and the control of the rate of stirring or agitation, as applicable.

IVRT Membrane Qualification: Membrane inertness should be evaluated in relation to membrane binding of the drug in the receptor solution (at a concentration relevant to the average concentration of the drug in the receptor solution at the end of the test). The recovery of the drug in solution is recommended to be within the range of 100% ± 5% at the end of the test duration to qualify the inertness of the membrane.

IVRT Receptor Solution Qualification: The composition of the receptor solution utilised for the IVRT study should be justified and the minimum solubility of drug in the IVRT receptor solution should be empirically determined in triplicate with the drug dissolved to saturation in the receptor solution, to a concentration exceeding the highest sample concentration obtained in the pivotal IVRT study, ideally by an order of magnitude or demonstrably sufficient to facilitate the linearity of the release rate for the duration of the study.

IVRT Receptor Solution Sampling Qualification: The accuracy and precision of receptor solution sample collection at each time point should be appropriately qualified.

IVRT Receptor Solution Sample Analytical Method Validation: The receptor sample HPLC analysis procedures should be validated in a manner compatible with the current FDA Guidance for Industry on Bioanalytical Method Validation, and/or the ICH Harmonised Tripartite Guideline on Validation of Analytical Procedures Q2 (R1). The validation of the receptor sample analytical method should include relevant qualifications of dilution integrity, as well as stability assessments with the highest relevant temperature in the receptor solution, which may be warmer than 32°C, for the duration of the IVRT study (e.g., 34°C for 6 hours).

IVRT Environmental Control: Ambient laboratory temperature and humidity during the study should be monitored and reported. An environmentally controlled temperature range of 21°C ± 2°C and a humidity range of 50% ± 20% relative humidity are recommended.

IVRT Linearity and Range: The linearity (r^2 value) of the release rate (slope) may be calculated across the range of the sampling times, which corresponds to the IVRT study duration. Linearity may be compared within and across all IVRT runs, and a minimum r^2 value ≥ 0.90 across the IVRT study duration (time range) is recommended.

IVRT Precision and Reproducibility: The intra-run and inter-run precision and reproducibility may be compared for the release rate (slopes) calculated for each diffusion cell. The mean, standard deviation, and percent coefficient of variation (%CV) among slopes may be calculated within and across all runs, and a minimum intra-run and inter-run %CV $\leq 15\%$ is recommended. Runs may be organised to facilitate simultaneous evaluation of intra/inter-instrumentation and/or intra/inter-operator precision and reproducibility.

IVRT Recovery, Mass Balance, and Dose Depletion: The recovery of the released drug in the receptor solution may be characterised in each diffusion cell as the accumulated amount of drug in the receptor solution over the IVRT duration. This may be expressed as a percentage of the amount of drug in the applied dose. The average dose depletion may thereby be estimated and should be reported, although the relevance of this at an infinite dose is questionable.

IVRT Discrimination in Sensitivity, Specificity, and Selectivity: The IVRT method should be able to discriminate drug release rates from similar formulations. For example, this may be evaluated by comparing the release rate from one product at 5% w/w drug with two comparable formulations in which the drug concentration has been altered – one with a higher strength (e.g., 7.5%), and one with a lower strength (e.g., 2.5%). Alternatives could be the manipulation of CQAs associated with the formulation being tested.

IVRT Robustness: The IVRT method may be considered robust to a variation in the test method if the average slope of that IVRT run (under altered conditions) is within ±15% of the average slope of the Precision and Reproducibility IVRT runs. Robustness testing may encompass variations in the IVRT method that are relevant to the apparatus and test method, for example:

a. Temperature variations (e.g., −1°C and +1°C relative to 32°C ± 1°C)
b. Dose volume variations (e.g., +10% and −10% in the dose volume)
c. Receptor solution variations (e.g., change in composition and/or pH)
d. Mixing rate variation (e.g., differences in stirring speed, or without stirring)

A Pivotal IVRT Study: In an IVRT pivotal study, it is generally accepted that for two products (Reference-R and Test-T) being tested, they should be dosed in an alternating sequence on successive diffusion cells. This approach helps ensure an unbiased comparison in the event of a systematic difference between runs. The assessment of the drug release from the test formulations (n=6 repetitions per formulation; Stage 1 only) should be performed based on the principles of the FDA's SUPAC-SS guidelines (Stage 1 only), the USP 40 <1724> (Semi-solid products-performance testing), and on recent guidelines released by the FDA. As common testing artefacts, such as air bubbles and membrane defects, can produce measurements that are not normally distributed, these guidelines recommend that a non-parametric statistical technique is used to evaluate the test results. For example, the Mann–Whitney U test is used to calculate the 90% confidence interval for the ratio of the slopes between the test and the reference products. In essence, the individual amounts of the drug released from the reference product (R) are plotted versus the square root of time and the resulting slopes are determined, providing the reference slopes. The process is repeated for the test product (T). The T/R slope ratios are calculated for each test-to-reference slope. After the T/R ratios have been calculated, they are ordered from the lowest to the highest. The 8th and 29th T/R ratios are identified and converted to percent (multiplied by 100). These values represent the 90% confidence interval for the ratio of test to reference release rates. To pass first stage testing, those ratios must be within the range of 75–133.33%. If the results do not meet this criterion, 4 additional tests of 6 cells should be performed, resulting in 12 additional slope determinations for each product tested. The T/R slope ratios for all 18 slopes for each product tested are determined. All 324 individual T/R slope ratios are ordered from the lowest to the highest. To pass this second stage testing, the 110th and 215th slope ratios, representing the 90% confidence interval, must be within the range of 75–133.33%. However, some regulatory agencies are now seeking to amend the ranges for Stages 1 and II to 90–110%.

6.3 *IN VITRO* (*EX VIVO*) DRUG PERMEATION AND PENETRATION TESTING (IVPT)

IVRT methodologies will only assess and compare the release of a drug from a formulation, and provide no insight on the ability of a drug to partition in and permeate across the stratum corneum and subsequent skin layers, nor any mechanistic understanding of how a formulation will affect the barrier properties of the skin (e.g., the effect of a penetration enhancer). Given the difficulties, costs, and time associated with *in vivo* experimentation, most topical and transdermal formulators attempt to use *ex vivo* methodology in order to optimise and compare formulations. IVPT is an established methodology, recognised by regulators, to assess the skin permeation (and in some cases, penetration) of a drug from topical or transdermal formulations. Such models are used to understand the influence of formulation on drug absorption across, and into the skin, whilst also being used to optimise and compare formulations during the early stages of development and through product development to post-marketing studies and competitor analysis.

Like IVRT, a typical IVPT method for topical and transdermal dosage forms is based on an open chamber diffusion cell system, such as a flow-through or static/Franz cell system in which a skin membrane is mounted. The test product (infinite or finite dose) is placed on the upper side of the skin in the open donor chamber of the diffusion cell and a receptor solution kept at a controlled temperature is either perfused with a continuous flow or placed on the other side of the skin. Permeation of drug from the topical or transdermal product through the membrane is monitored by assay of sequentially collected samples from the receptor fluid whilst the drug in the different skin layers can also be recovered and assayed. These samples can be collected either manually or automated depending on the system employed. As a result of the often low levels of the drug permeating into the receiver solution and into the skin, highly sensitive analytical methods (e.g., HPLC or LC-MS/MS) tends to be the analytical method of choice. A plot of the amount of the drug permeating the skin per unit area ($\mu g/cm^2$) against time yields a permeation profile from which a lag phase and pseudo steady-state flux can be determined (see Chapter 2). A mass balance where the amount of the drug (as absolute amounts or % of applied dose) in the different skin layers and that retained elsewhere in the system (skin surface, left in diffusion cell, evaporated, etc.) can also be performed. In addition, if the drug being assessed has a suitable label or chromophore, then drug deposition in the skin can be visualised using autoradiography, fluorescence/confocal microscopy, Raman microscopy, and, in some cases, histology.

The following describes some of the key experimental variables and risks associated with IVPT and how they can be mitigated.

6.3.1   THE CHOICE OF MEMBRANE

It has long been established that excised human skin is the "gold standard" for *in vitro/ex vivo* permeation studies, as it can give a good approximation to the *in vivo* situation. Human skin samples can be obtained from a variety of sources, including from skin banks or by donation from a patient undergoing a surgical procedure, such as an abdominoplasty or breast reduction. However, in most cases, the investigator has little control over the preoperative handling of the skin membrane until excision. For example, prior to surgical procedures, it is common for the skin to be swabbed to remove microorganisms and hence minimise the potential for infection of the surgical wound. Typically, such disinfectants are alcoholic, which can extract lipids from the stratum corneum, thus altering the barrier properties of the membrane, and may also contain other potentially damaging chemicals such as cetrimide. Further, if tissues are obtained from skin banks, then the material will have been stored for a period of time prior to packaging and shipping to the investigator. Clearly, additional processing of the membrane increases the risk of damage to, or degradation of, the tissue. A concern with experiments using skin donated from a particular surgical procedure arises from the use of skin from one body site, or from one sex and age range. As described in Chapter 1 (Section 1.3.3), variations in skin permeability are evident between different body sites and it is thus unrealistic to expect that tissue samples obtained from, for example, breast reduction surgery or from scalp punch biopsies would give the same permeation characteristics. Often the investigator has little choice in which site the skin is from, but in such cases, some caution must be attached to data obtained on a membrane from a site that is different to that for drug delivery or hazard evaluation. If experiments are designed to simply rank a series of formulations, then the history and site of the tissue may not be of great importance. However, for most experimental situations, where fundamental drug flux data is sought, or when experiments are designed to mimic the *in vivo* situation, then knowledge of the tissue history is important to avoid misinterpretation of data.

There are ethical and legal constraints to obtaining and using human material, and this has led many investigators to turn to alternative models. Non-human primate skin is a potential alternative but this is usually more difficult source than human skin. Pig skin is accepted as the animal model most closely resembling human skin; the stratum corneum of the pig is similar in thickness to the human membrane, and although pig skin lipid content does vary to that of human tissue, it has remarkably similar permeability properties. Penetration enhancer effects also appear to be well-predicted by this model membrane, which has an added advantage in that it may be relatively easy to acquire. However, as with the human tissue, there are variations in the permeability properties of pig skin with body site. Alternative animal membranes all have significant limitations and any data produced must be treated with caution as there is very little, if any, evidence that data from, for example, rodent skin, can be translated to the clinical setting. For example, although hairless mouse has been widely used by numerous workers, it differs markedly to human tissue. In terms of structure, the lipid content of hairless mouse stratum corneum is greater than that in human skin, and the rodent tissue is somewhat thinner. In diffusional terms, hairless mouse tissue loses its integrity rapidly whereas the human stratum corneum barrier remains intact for longer periods of time, and many researchers report that the hairless mouse skin is thus an unacceptable model for predicting human skin permeation. Alternative rodent models have been selected to mimic human skin diffusional behaviour, which include hairless rat skin and guinea pig skin, neither of which appear to be any more relevant than hairless mouse.

It is readily apparent from the above that there can be some difficulties associated with using human skin for permeation studies, and that these can be exacerbated by using animal membranes. One approach that has been suggested to overcome these issues is the use of reconstituted or reconstructed human epidermis (RHE) membranes which are ready-to-use, highly differentiated 3D tissue models consisting of normal, human-derived epidermal keratinocytes cultured at an air–liquid interface on specially prepared tissue culture inserts. RHE exhibit human epidermal tissue structure and cellular morphology with greater uniformity and reproducibility. The 3D structure, consisting of organised and proliferative basal cells, spinous and granular layers, and cornified epidermal layers, are mitotically and metabolically active. Such RHE membranes are used throughout industry in formulation development, toxicity (irritation and corrosivity) testing, disease (mechanistic) modelling, barrier repair, and metabolism studies However, at present, the generation of an intact stratum corneum membrane in the RHE with the same permeability characteristics as that found *in vivo* is proving difficult (along with a lack of appendages); RHEs are typically around ten times more permeable to drug transport than excised human tissue.

Various synthetic artificial model membranes have also been employed for permeation studies. Such membranes generally comprise lipids supported on a solid inert matrix in which the lipid element is intended to mimic the intercellular lipid domain of the stratum corneum. Whilst the lipid content can be modified to better mimic human skin permeation, and excipients such as penetration enhancers can be added to the lipid matrix to examine effects on membrane diffusivity or partitioning phenomena, these solid supported liquid/semi-solid membranes tend to be relatively unstable to formulation components which can limit their use. More structured lipid matrices have also been prepared to mimic the barrier properties of the lipid domains within stratum corneum. Thus, lamellar sheets can be obtained by fusion of liposomes onto a solid supporting membrane. The liposomes can be prepared from simple lipid mixtures, or can contain lipids that are found within human stratum corneum.

A relatively recent development is the Strat-M™ synthetic membrane which is described as being constructed of two layers of polyethersulfone (PES, more resistant to diffusion) on top of one layer of polyolefin (more open and permeable). These polymeric layers create a porous structure with a gradient across the membrane in terms of pore size and diffusivity. The porous structure is impregnated with a proprietary blend of synthetic lipids, imparting additional skin-like properties to the synthetic membrane. The manufacturers claim that permeation through Strat-M correlates closely to human skin. It should be noted that most of the data to support this correlation was conducted with approved topical drugs with ideal physiochemical properties rather than novel agents or formulations.

More simplistic model membranes have also been used in drug delivery and hazard evaluation studies. Artificial "chemical" membranes offer the advantages of reproducibility and control – the membrane is isotropic, there is no regional variability, and permeation can be described by simple mathematical rules. The most common example of this is probably polydimethylsiloxane (silastic or PDMS) membrane which provides a "non-porous" hydrophobic reproducible barrier. However, whilst usually described as a "hydrophobic non-porous membrane", it is important to note that the membrane does allow passage of water – equivalent to a transepidermal water loss – during permeation studies. Such a simple membrane has been used in formulation optimisation studies and for testing physicochemical principles. Nevertheless, clearly the simplicity of such membranes has disadvantages in terms of poorly representing human tissue *in vivo* – no metabolism, minimal variability, lack of lipid domains, simple permeation processes rather than the more complex multiple processes occurring in the heterogeneous human skin, no shunt routes, et cetera. Complexity can be built into artificial membranes to overcome some of the above issues, but the membranes remain a simplistic representation of a highly complex biological organ.

6.3.2   THE CHOICE OF MEMBRANE LAYER AND ITS PREPARATION

The above described the types of skin models available, but one further question remains when selecting either human or animal skin for *in vitro* permeation experiments: which skin layers should be used? One of the most widely used membranes is epidermal tissue, comprising the nucleate epidermis and the overlying stratum corneum. The rationale for using this membrane is that the stratum corneum provides the major barrier to permeation of most penetrants, and hence the viable epidermis, which is essentially an aqueous medium, merely provides mechanical support to the stratum corneum. In addition, the capillaries removing traversed molecules from the skin are found at the epidermal–dermal junction within skin *in vivo*, and hence the dermis does not usually contribute as a significant barrier to the permeation of most drugs. Although there are sometimes good scientific reasons for selecting an isolated stratum corneum membrane for permeation experiments, such as mechanistic evaluation or to increase drug levels in the receptor compartment for ease of sample analysis, this membrane is fragile and easily damaged, and so membrane integrity checks before and after the permeation experiment are essential. As the dermis can also be regarded as essentially an aqueous support medium, then "full thickness" membranes can also be selected. These membranes contain all the skin layers (stratum corneum, nucleate epidermis, and the dermis) but they can be cumbersome, as the dermal tissue is relatively thick compared with the outer skin layers. As an alternative, dermatomed membranes or "split thickness" can be obtained of varying thicknesses to provide a sample that comprises the stratum corneum, nucleate epidermis, and upper dermis.

It can be argued that the appropriate membrane to select depends on the nature of the permeant under investigation and the question being asked. For compounds that are hydrophilic, then the barrier to permeation largely resides within the stratum corneum intercellular lipid domains, and hence the presence of essentially aqueous viable epidermal cells or dermal material will not significantly affect the diffusional process; permeated drugs will clear easily and readily into the (aqueous) receptor phase. However, for highly lipophilic molecules, then the presence of the "aqueous" barrier provided by the viable epidermis/dermis can be significant depending on the drugs site of action. In these cases, where the permeant log octanol/water partition coefficient tends to be above 3, the use of dermatomed skin membranes can significantly retard clearance of the molecules from the membrane into the receptor phase, and so the viable epidermis alone may be more appropriate. However, neither of the above takes into account any binding (or metabolism if the skin retains its viability) of the drug that may occur in the different skin layers and, as such, dermatomed skin is often the membrane of choice for permeation studies.

There are several well-established methods for the preparation of skin membranes. Most commonly, excised tissue samples (e.g., from surgery or skin banks) are further processed to provide the desired membranes. Typically, excess fatty and connective tissue is removed from the skin samples before storage. Samples can be stored frozen, and whilst some authors report that incorporation of cryo-protectants may be beneficial, others claim that using, for example, glycerol can modify the permeability characteristics of the tissue. Methods for preparing dermatomed membranes from excised skin samples vary between investigators but clearly involve the use of a dermatome set at a required thickness and, for ease of manipulation, cutting skin partially frozen at the surface. The most common method for the preparation of epidermal membranes (nucleate epidermis plus stratum corneum) is that of heat separation as first proposed by Kligman and Christophers (1963). The skin sample, trimmed of excess fatty and connective tissue, is immersed in 60°C water for ca. 45 seconds. The skin is then pinned, dermal side down and the epidermal membrane can be peeled off from the underlying dermis, having been split by the warm water. The "peeling" again requires practice and can be done with a pair of blunt forceps, rounded tweezers, or with a gloved finger; the latter being the approach that generally minimises stratum corneum damage. The same membrane can then be used to obtain the stratum corneum by floating the resultant viable epidermal membrane with the stratum corneum uppermost (i.e., not in direct contact with the enzyme) on a solution of trypsin. The enzyme digests the viable tissue that can thus be removed by swabbing and rinsing in fresh aqueous media. The fragile stratum corneum membranes can then be floated onto a mesh (polytetrafluoroethylene [PTFE]-coated) where the membranes can be air and desiccator dried for storage. Use of a PTFE mesh allows easy removal of the membranes when dry, or if used wet.

6.3.3 The Choice of Diffusion Cell

The two most basic types of diffusion cells used to assess topical penetration/permeation are either a static version, originally pioneered by Tom Franz (Franz cell), or flow-through systems developed by Robert Bronaugh (Bronaugh flow-through cell) and others. Both static and flow-through diffusion cells (Figure 6.2). are similar in concept, where a membrane (synthetic or biological) is positioned between a donor chamber and a receptor chamber which is kept at a controlled temperature (via a water bath or jacket, usually at 37°C to maintain surface skin temperature at 32°C as an *in vivo* mimic). The main difference between the two systems is within the design of the receptor chamber for the receptor fluid which serves as a reservoir for drugs as they permeate through the membrane (as described below).

Most simply, static diffusion cells tend to be upright and made of glass, with the donor compartment available for application of the permeant and the receptor compartment of a fixed volume containing receptor fluid. The receptor fluid is agitated, most commonly with a magnetic bar stirrer, and a portal from the receptor compartment allows removal of receptor fluid at required time intervals. They are versatile in that the diffusional area can easily be modified (typically from 0.5 to 5 cm²), the receptor volume can be changed to "concentrate", the permeant to facilitate analysis (around 1 to 20 mL) and the donor compartment can be covered to mimic occlusive application of formulations to skin, or left open if appropriate. These cells are thus widely used for evaluating drug uptake into skin, finite dose permeation, or steady state flux of a drug either alone or in formulations – the relatively large and open donor compartment allows simple application of semi-solid formulations or transdermal patch formulations to the skin surface. A limitation of this type of cell can be the need to add organic or biological solvents (ethanol, polyethylene glycol oleyl ether, surfactant, serum albumin, etc.) to ensure sink conditions are met in the receiver fluid and ensure that permeant solubility in the receptor solution is not rate-determining to drug flux. This is particularly important when evaluating flux of more lipophilic drugs. Added solvents in the receiving fluid can themselves migrate into the membrane or tissue and create artificial environments that are not present *in vivo*. This may not be material if the intent is to rank compounds or formulations; however, when the information will be used to accurately assess penetration or permeation, then their inclusion should be avoided. Some biological "solvents" (e.g., serum albumin) can also cause analytical difficulties and may require additional sample processing that can result in loss of drug or inaccurate values. When assessing water-soluble compounds, saline, or buffer solutions, or deionised (DI) water should be sufficient for maintaining sink conditions, but this needs to be confirmed during method development. Another limitation of the static diffusion cells is the necessity for manual sampling, which can make sampling of certain time points (middle of the night) difficult.

In contrast to the static cells, flow-through diffusion cells attempt to mimic *in vivo* conditions with a flow-through receptor chamber to mimic the blood supply, and with an unstirred donor phase equivalent to a drug formulation. In common with the static systems, flow-through diffusion cells have temperature control, and most allow various formulation applications (occlusive or open application, finite or infinite dosing). However, there are some differences between the static and flow-through systems that can be important in some cases. The continuous flow of receptor solution beneath the diffusion cell (typically around 1 to 2 mL/h) theoretically ensures sink conditions are maintained throughout the diffusion experiment without the need of any additional solvent; however, this may not be the case with highly lipophilic compounds (logP >4), which can be undetectable in the receiving fluid despite extremely sensitive analytical methods. Nevertheless, the flow of the receptor solution under the skin membrane causes turbulence that effectively stirs the receptor compartment and minimises the boundary layer underneath the membrane, whereas with static cells, even with a bar stirrer, there can be a stagnant layer underneath the membrane. Various designs of flow-through apparatus exist, with various levels of "automation" which makes difficult sampling points (middle of the night) more amenable.

A recent example of an improved flow-through cell is known as "MedFlux-HT®", which is a continuous flow system with a carefully designed flowpath to enhance local clearance of the receiver solution from beneath human skin. This design allows the user to generate more accurate and more detailed flux profiles within a shorter time frame. The increased local clearance from beneath the skin and optimised receiver fluid flow improves sink conditions and facilitates the analysis of lipophilic compounds which has been previously problematic. In addition, MedFlux-HT has been engineered with an in-built high-throughput approach to sample collection and analysis. The system is thermostatically controlled to maintain constant physiological temperature and the collection of the receiver fluid is automated for higher throughput sample quantification. The MedFlux-HT system also minimises the amount of skin required for dosing, allowing greater numbers of replicates from an often limited tissue supply.

6.3.4 FORMULATION APPLICATION CONSIDERATIONS

It is difficult to generalise protocols for application of the drug during *in vitro* studies since these are dependent on the experimental rationale. For example, protocols designed to examine the risks associated with occupational exposure to a small amount of a volatile solvent spilt on the skin will differ to protocols examining permeation of oestradiol from a patch applied to the skin for five days, which will differ again from analysing the effect of formulation metamorphosis upon application over a few hours.

In general terms, when an infinite dose is applied to the tissue, it is inherently assumed that there is no change in the drug concentration (or more accurately in its thermodynamic activity) during the experiment and that there is no formulation metamorphosis upon application. Clearly, this assumption is not valid when, for example, a defined permeant concentration is used since some drug molecules will traverse the skin and volatile components of a formulation will evaporate, irrespective of the amounts applied. To minimise the errors of donor solution depletion, some researchers use saturated drug solutions and incorporate small amounts of solid material that will dissolve and so replenish permeant molecules that have crossed the membrane. This approach has in itself the assumption that the rate of permeant dissolution from the solid is as rapid as the movement of molecules through the membrane, but the use of excess solid permeant within the donor does give some confidence that the dose remains infinite. Generally, if the permeant concentration in the donor phase does not fall by more than 10% from saturation during the experimental period, then infinite dosing can reasonably be assumed. In contrast, a finite dose (2–10 mg/cm² depending upon formulation type) is expected to deplete on the skin surface and demonstrate, to some extent, formulation metamorphosis (generation of a residual phase on the skin surface). In general terms, experimental conditions including application dosages, exposure times and procedures should mimic as closely as possible the *in vivo* situation to provide appropriate data.

When studying the ability of a drug to permeate the skin per se, the choice of vehicle in which to apply the drug can also vary depending on the experimental rationale. For example, if wanting to examine the fundamental permeation behaviour of a molecule, then a simple aqueous-based solvent/solvent system/vehicle with adequate drug solubility is preferable. However, often the permeant will be lipophilic and hence will have a low aqueous solubility; with a low aqueous solubility, the potential for donor depletion during an experiment increases, especially as the lipophilic permeant will traverse the tissue relatively easily. Consequently, researchers often choose alternative vehicles such as water/alcohol mixtures or propylene glycol, but these vehicles may interact with the structure and barrier function of the stratum corneum to promote drug flux and so can confound the results, especially when screening a number of drug candidates to select one for formulation development. An inert universal solvent system for drug candidate screening is yet to be demonstrated. Nevertheless, when selecting a vehicle for permeation studies, it is important to ensure that the vehicle does not interact with the membrane, or that if it does affect the structure or integrity of the membrane, then appropriate control experiments (e.g., using the same vehicle for comparison of different formulations) are undertaken. Interactions between the drug and the vehicle or between the drug and other excipients in the formulation can also modify the permeation behaviour of the penetrant and needs to be considered.

As previously stated in Chapter 2 (Section 2.4.4), the degree of ionisation of a permeant can affect the amounts of the material that traverses the stratum corneum membrane; the pH-partition hypothesis states that ions would permeate through the lipoidal matrix slower than the uncharged species. However, as aqueous vehicles are often used in permeation studies, it is feasible that the flux of an ionised species could be greater than that of its un-ionised parent, since the flux is the product of permeability coefficient (low for ion, high for un-ionised species) and the concentration (high for ion, low for un-ionised species). When using ionisable drugs in topical and transdermal delivery studies, it is clearly important to understand the level of drug ionisation and the impact on the drug's solubility and stability in the vehicle and its ability to permeate the skin. In short, do not assume, test!

6.3.5 PERMEANT DETECTION

Experimental design can be influenced by the method of detection for the permeant traversing through the membrane. Most commonly, chromatographic methods such as LC-MS/MS, HPLC, or ultra-performance liquid chromatography (UPLC) are selected for analysing the permeant in the receptor fluid, or in extracts (washings) of the membrane. Chromatographic methodologies have significant advantages over other methods of detection/analysis in that the methods are versatile and can be adapted to many or most permeants traversing the skin by appropriate selection of columns, mobile phases, and detectors. In addition, multiple components from formulations permeating through the membrane can be analysed simultaneously and the methods currently available are relatively rapid and easy to use (for example, using auto-sample injectors). Importantly, from analysis of retention times, chromatographic methods measure what species has actually come through the membrane rather than what species was placed onto the membrane; biotransformations (metabolism) can occur during permeation through viable skin. One disadvantage with chromatographic methods (especially HPLC) arises as a result of the relatively low amounts of the drug permeating across the skin which can lead to problems with accurate detection and quantification, especially when components of the skin can interfere with the analysis. Methods are available to remove such contamination from the samples, for example, using pre-columns, solid phase extraction columns, solvent precipitation, or reconstitution. However, such further sample preparation can introduce errors within the analysis.

One approach to avoid these above problems is to use radiolabelled permeants. A variety of labels can be employed, but most common are tritium (H^3) and carbon 14 (C^{14}). As detection is by scintillation counting, there are few restrictions on using large receptor volumes taken from diffusion cells, analysis is rapid and generally automated, and very low concentrations of permeants can be detected with a high degree of accuracy. One major constraint on the use of radiolabelled permeants is the stability of the label employed. For example, tritium exchange is a real problem where the tritium located on the drug is exchanged with hydrogen on water molecules, resulting in water flux being measured rather than the drug itself. Clearly the flux of water through skin is greater than that expected for most drugs or hazardous agents, and hence falsely elevated data for permeation will be recorded. To mitigate this risk, control experiments are required, such as the use of a radiochemical detector to ensure label stability, rather than just relying on a scintillation counter. Another method to check radiolabel integrity after a permeation study is to warm a sample of receptor fluid under vacuum; if the level of radioactivity diminishes as water evaporates, then tritium exchange has likely occurred. Another issue with isotopically labelled permeants is the restricted range of materials that may be studied – common therapeutic agents and hazardous materials can be purchased with a radiolabel, but more specialised chemicals are custom-synthesised with associated high cost. Further, it is clear that novel chemical agents being evaluated for delivery by the topical or transdermal route will not be available radiolabelled. Additional complications arise from the handling and storage of radioactive materials. When using radiolabelled permeants, it is important to prepare the donor solution appropriately. The permeant formulation will usually be prepared with "cold" (non-radiolabelled) permeant and then spiked with a very small amount "hot" (radiolabelled) material. If the spiking is after the formulation has been prepared, then appropriate mixing is required and the homogeneity of the label needs to be checked. In some cases, the thermodynamic activity of the drug pre- and post-addition of "hot" material may also need to be confirmed.

Spectroscopic methods have also been used to identify and quantify the amounts of materials traversing through membranes, and examples of such techniques include ATR-FTIR spectroscopy and Raman and confocal microscopy. The major limitations with such methods arise from interference of the skin itself and the limitations on the number of drugs that have the required spectrum for analysis without the use of some form of conjugate label which inherently will change the physicochemical properties of the drug in question and potentially invalidate the data produced. Bioassays can also be used for some large molecular weight drugs.

6.3.6   Donor Solution Concentration

In addition to the considerations outlined for permeant analysis or finite/infinite dose application, study design should also attend to the concentration (thermodynamic activity) of the permeant in the donor solution. As with most of the factors outlined above, the concentration of donor solutions will vary with the aim of the experiment. However, selecting a standard amount or concentration of differing drugs when comparing formulations can be misleading. As described earlier (Chapter 2, Section 2.5.2), it is the thermodynamic activity of the permeant in the vehicle that provides the driving force for permeation. By modifying vehicle components, the thermodynamic activity of the same concentration of material can change radically. For example, consider a drug with a solubility of 18 mg/g in propylene glycol and 180 mg/g in N-methylpyrrolidone (NMP). It would be erroneous to compare permeation of the drug from solutions of the two solvents each containing 18 mg/g of the drug, since the propylene glycol solution would be saturated, giving the maximum thermodynamic activity and hence maximal flux, whereas the NMP solution would be at ca. 10% saturated, and hence would deliver considerably less of the drug. Clearly for formulation comparisons, it is preferable to compare fluxes where the permeant is at the same thermodynamic activity in both formulations, most easily achieved by maintaining permeant saturation in both formulations, or selecting the same fraction of saturation. The influence of thermodynamic activity in contrast to concentration gradients was illustrated in Chapter 2 (Section 2.5.2).

6.3.7   Receptor Solution

Ideally, the receptor (also commonly termed "receiver") solution used for *in vitro* permeation experiments should mimic as closely as possible the *in vivo* situation. As described in Chapter 1 (Section 1.2.2), the dermis contains the cutaneous microvasculature and lymph vessels that readily remove chemicals which have crossed the stratum corneum and viable epidermal layers, thus maintaining sink conditions for permeation (i.e., the concentration gradient across the membrane is maximal). The selection of an appropriate receptor solution to mimic this highly efficient removal of permeant is thus essential for good *in vitro* experimental design. In practice, ensuring that the concentration of the permeating species does not exceed 10% of its solubility in the receptor solution is usually sufficient to ensure that the flux of material through the skin is not significantly slowed by modification of the concentration gradient across the membrane. The selection of a receiver solution largely depends on the nature of the permeant and on diffusion cell design. Flow-through systems generally minimise the accumulation of permeant in the receptor and so allow the use of aqueous receptor media even for moderately lipophilic materials. With static systems, the potential for violating the "10% rule" is greater.

Aqueous receptor solutions are the most commonly used media for hydrophilic and moderately lipophilic (up to a log P octanol/water of around 2) permeants. Buffered solutions, such as phosphate, around pH 7.4 are often used where species are ionisable. For un-ionisable species, water may be used and to the receptor solutions, an antimicrobial agent may be added. Difficulties arise when the permeant is much more lipophilic or where aqueous solubility of the permeant is low. Such permeants are well cleared *in vivo*, and so a more appropriate receptor solution is required. Consequently, many researchers investigating permeation of lipophilic materials add solubilising agents to the receptor medium. Common examples include the addition of surfactants (e.g., between 1.5 and 20% Volpo N20, or 1.5 to 6% Triton X-100 added to the aqueous receptor fluid), protein (e.g., adding 3% bovine serum albumin), or the use of an organic solvent as a component of the receptor solution. For many studies, this latter option has been the most popular and a wide composition of ethanol/water co-solvent systems has been used. Typically, 25% ethanol/water receiver phases have been shown to provide reasonable sink conditions for many lipophilic molecules traversing the skin.

Whilst it is essential to select an appropriate receptor solution to ensure clearance of the permeant, it is also important to consider the effects of the receptor on the barrier properties of the skin. Thus, when using a solubilising agent in the receiver fluid to increase permeant solubility, it is essential to ensure that the solubilising agent does not permeabilise or damage the skin, since several common solubilisers are also chemical penetration enhancers (see Chapter 3). This is particularly evident when adding surfactants, or if significant levels of ethanol are introduced into the medium. Indeed, even moderate levels of ethanol in the receptor phase (e.g., up to 25%) have caused some workers some concerns; membrane integrity may be compromised. It should also be borne in mind that components of a receptor phase are also potential permeants that can diffuse "backwards" from a more concentrated solution (the receptor fluid) through the skin membrane and into the donor phase. Thus, if an aqueous formulation has been applied to the membrane surface, permeation of ethanol from the receptor phase back into the donor phase is possible, which can alter the applied formulation and hence permeation characteristics in terms of, for example, modification of the thermodynamic activity of the drug in the formulation.

6.3.8   INTEGRITY CHECKS

As the preparation of skin membranes is a complex process, there is considerable scope for damaging the tissue. In addition, the skin could also be diseased or damaged prior to removal or separation. There are numerous proposed methods to verify the integrity of membranes used for *in vitro* permeation studies. One approach is to monitor the permeation of a well-known compound through the skin prior to (and/or after) examining the test material. For these studies, tritiated water or radiolabelled glucose/sucrose/mannitol have been all been used, but have the limitations previously identified in Section 6.3.5. Full permeation profiles (and associated flux) can be obtained, or alternatively, a single time point of permeation for such markers. Criteria used to reject skin with permeability coefficients differing to this "norm" are rather arbitrary. For example, some researchers use criteria for a particular skin sample that is based on the resultant marker data fitting in a specified range, whilst others accept skin samples based on the marker data being within a specified number of standard deviations of the mean.

An alternative approach to assess membrane integrity has been to measure trans-epidermal water loss (TEWL) prior to experimentation. This has the advantage of not applying materials to the membrane to check integrity, but again is a measure of water traversing the tissue that may not directly correlate with permeation pathways for lipophilic materials. Likewise, electrical resistance of skin membranes can be used as an integrity check, but value of such techniques post-formulation application is extremely questionable, especially as formulations are often designed to increase skin permeability to allow for enhanced drug permeation. More simply, an aliquot of the receptor solution placed onto the surface of the membrane can monitor gross skin integrity – if holes are present in the membrane, then the liquid will rapidly be lost from the surface. This becomes even more obvious if a dye is included. Other methods include the "eye-balling" or statistical analysis of data produced in order to reject "obvious" or statistically verified outliers. Nevertheless, because of the above difficulties in ensuring tissue integrity, and considering the inherent variability within human skin permeability, it is absolutely critical to ensure that sufficient replicate experiments are performed to justify the conclusions derived; this often includes a large number of skin donors and sufficient replicates within each skin donor (see Section 6.3.11).

6.3.9 Temperature

It is well known that skin permeability varies with temperature, especially at temperatures beyond the melting points of stratum corneum bilayer lipids. Thus, most topical and transdermal drug delivery experiments are performed with a skin surface temperature of 32°C to mirror the *in vivo* situation. This is generally achieved by maintaining the receptor fluid at around 37°C with the cells either jacketed, or immersed in a water bath or heat block at the appropriate temperature. The skin surface temperature can then be monitored/verified using temperature probes placed on the stratum corneum or a calibrated thermal camera to ensure the receiver fluid temperature of 37°C, is achieving a skin surface temperature of 32°C ± 2°C. Nevertheless, the temperature required is often cell type specific and it is always advisable to measure skin temperature to ensure it mimics *in vivo* conditions.

6.3.10 Experimental Duration

In vitro permeation experiments can vary in duration from a matter of minutes to days. For finite dose studies of occupational exposure to a hazardous material, it may be appropriate to expose the membrane to the permeant for seconds before washing off and monitoring the amounts traversing the membrane. In contrast, if examining the delivery of drug from a once a week patch formulation, then clearly permeation is monitored for at least seven days.

Experimental duration should consider several factors. Firstly, membrane integrity must be maintained throughout the experimental period. This will vary with the membrane being employed – clearly artificial membranes are generally more robust than are biological tissues. Secondly, if assessing pseudo steady-state flux of a permeant, it is often advised that the experiment run for a time period greater than 2.7 times the lag time – steady-state conditions are not attained until this period. Thirdly, the experimental duration may depend on the permeant assay sensitivity; poor permeants with difficult assays need to run long enough to allow permeation of sufficient material for detection and analysis.

6.3.11   IN VITRO EXPERIMENT REPLICATES

Due to the variability in permeation data between and within skin samples, statistical validity for the data can only be claimed where sufficient replicates have been performed. Typically, when just screening formulations, a minimum of 5–6 replicates on one skin donor may give the rank order required. However, when trying to relate the data derived to the *in vivo* setting, then a more robust study is required. For such studies, between three and six replicates per skin donor with a minimum of three skin donors have been proposed. In addition, testing different formulations on the same donor skin (again with replicates), allows a direct comparison of product performance, whilst normalising the natural variation in skin permeability between different donors; taking the ratio of flux or enhancement in this way allows each piece of skin to act as its own control. More recent guidelines (Acyclovir cream draft guidance [see Section 6.3.14]) have suggested that a pilot study be performed to assess the variability in permeability between donors' values in order to derive the number of skin donors and replicates required for statistically meaningful data.

6.3.12   MASS BALANCE

Further confidence in the validity of permeation data can be obtained by determining the mass balance (or total recovery) of permeant at the end of the experiment. In addition to the amount of permeant analysed in the receptor solution, washing from the skin surface, from the donor and receptor chambers of the diffusion cell, from any covering on top of the cell when occlusion is used (e.g., coverslips or Parafilm), and amounts of permeant present in the membrane (obtained by extraction with solvents or using a tissue solubiliser) can all be recorded. In general, mass balances of a minimum of 90% are required to be able to interpret the data in any meaningful way. It is often difficult to get mass balances beyond 90% using non-radiolabelled compounds. If considering mass balance studies where the drug is to be quantified on the surface and tape strips, it is critical to ensure the solvent systems are capable of extracting the drug from the different formulation types and tape. Oil-based formulations such as ointments are particularly challenging. It is not uncommon to see lower recoveries (50–80%) when these types of formulations are examined.

6.3.13   EXPRESSION OF RESULTS

When permeability data have been obtained from infinitely dosed steady state experiments, then a flux or permeability coefficient (flux = permeability coefficient × donor concentration) can be reported (see Chapter 2, Section 2.5.1). Where steady state has not been achieved, or where experimental data points are insufficient to quote a rate, then the amount traversing in a given time period may be used.

For finite dose applications, generally steady-state flux is not obtained and a rate of absorption over a given time period can be reported (see Chapter 2, Section 2.5.3). Alternatively, data from finite dose experiments can report a pseudo steady-state flux or the amount or percentage of applied dose permeated at a given time period. Other clinically relevant values that are often reported from finite dose studies are the maximum flux obtained and the time taken to reach the maximum flux. Alternatively, the amount absorbed at each time point can be plotted against time and an area under the curve (AUC) calculated. The vast majority of literature expresses permeation data in arithmetic terms – typically providing means and standard deviations for fluxes, permeability coefficients, et cetera. However, measurements such as peak flux, cumulative amount permeated, and pseudo steady-state flux are rarely normally distributed, often requiring the use of non-parametric tests to determine significance (e.g., Williams et al., 1992). Fortunately, evidence suggests that log transformation of these values yields a normal (Gaussian) distribution. Therefore, although data may be most easily presented in plain values, statistical analysis is best carried out on the base-10 log transformed values. This observation is reflected in the draft guidance released by the FDA.

6.3.14   PIVOTAL IVPT METHODOLOGICAL DESIGN

Having discussed some of the major factors to be considered when designing and performing *in vitro* permeation experiments, it is prudent to consider some of the major recommendations from regulatory bodies with regard to aspects of study design. Such regulatory guidelines are continually being modified and adapted, and are appropriate to particular sectors of activity – hazard evaluation of pesticides may require different protocols to bioequivalence testing of pharmaceutical formulations, which can differ to those needed for assessing cosmetic preparations. Protocol guidelines have been provided by (amongst others) the European Centre for the Validation of Alternative Methods (ECVAM), the European Cosmetic Toiletry and Perfumery Association (COLIPA), the European Centre for Ecotoxicology and Toxicology of Chemicals (ECETOC), the U.S. Food and Drug Administration (FDA), the U.S. Environmental Protection Agency (EPA), and the OECD (Organisation for Economic Co-operation and Development). However, at the time of writing the most up-to-date guidance can be taken from the FDA draft Guidance Document on Acyclovir cream which was revised in 2016 and which covers the development, calibration, qualification, validation, and performance of a pivotal IVPT study. It states pivotal study design should be a parallel, single-dose, multiple-replicate per treatment group study using excised human skin with a competent skin barrier mounted on a qualified diffusion cell system. Ideally, all formulations tested should be blinded and randomly assigned across the diffusion cells and skin donors. As an exemplar, the guidance is provided in more detail below:

Method Development
Dosing: A single, un-occluded dose in the range of 5–15 mg cream/cm^2 that is retained on the skin for the duration of the study is recommended. The amount actually used should be justified based on the formulation

type being investigated. Formulation metamorphosis or transition (residual phase) should be considered and ideally investigated.

Replicates: A minimum of four dosed replicates per donor per formulation is recommended, with the number of donors statistically justified (see later) from a pilot study.

Study duration/sampling: The study duration should be sufficient to characterise the cutaneous pharmacokinetics of the drug, including a sufficiently complete flux profile to identify the maximum (peak) flux and a decline in the flux thereafter across multiple subsequent time points. The sampling frequency should be selected to provide suitable resolution for the flux profile, and a minimum of eight non-zero sampling time points is recommended across the study duration (e.g., 24–48 hours). Information should be provided to support the selection of the IVPT apparatus, product dose amount, sampling times, stirring/flow rate, and other parameters of the test method.

Method Verification/Validation

The apparatus, methodologies, and study conditions utilised in the study should be appropriately validated and incorporate the following qualifications and controls:

Apparatus Qualification: Suitable apparatus for the method can include appropriate vertical diffusion cells and flow-through diffusion cells. The qualification of each diffusion cell should, at minimum, qualify the diffusional area of the orifice in which the skin is mounted, the volume of the receptor solution compartment in each diffusion cell, the control of a $32°C \pm 1°C$ temperature (at the skin surface throughout the study duration; measured by a calibrated infrared thermometer using a non-dosed control), and the control of the rate of stirring or flow rate, as applicable.

Skin Qualification: Excised human skin is recommended as the membrane for the study. The validity of each skin section dosed in the study should be qualified using an appropriate test procedure to evaluate the stratum corneum barrier integrity. Acceptable barrier integrity tests may be based upon tritiated water permeation, transepidermal water loss (TEWL), or electrical impedance/conductance measured across the skin. The test parameters and acceptance criteria utilised for the skin barrier integrity test should be justified. The skin thickness should be measured and reported for each skin section and should be consistent for all donors whose skin is included in the study. The assignment of replicate skin sections from a donor to each treatment group should be randomised, as feasible. Control of the skin before and during the study is obviously extremely important, which includes the skin storage conditions (e.g., duration for which the skin was frozen) and the number of freeze-thaw cycles to which the skin was exposed before use and the preparation of the skin (e.g., dermatoming of skin sections) and the thickness of skin sections mounted on the diffusion cells. Skin from the same anatomical location should be utilised from all donors, and the demographics (age, race, sex) should be reported for all donors.

Receptor Solution Qualification: The composition and pH of the receptor solution utilised for the study should be qualified in relation to its compatibility with the skin as well as the solubility and stability of the drug(s) being studied. The minimum solubility of the drug in the receptor solution should be empirically determined in triplicate with drug dissolved to saturation in the receptor solution, to a concentration exceeding the highest sample concentration in the pivotal study, ideally by an order of magnitude. Strategies to improve the solubility of drug in the receptor solution that may have the potential to alter the permeability of the skin are not recommended. The inclusion of an antimicrobial agent in the receptor solution (e.g., ~0.1% sodium azide or ~0.01% gentamicin sulfate) is an approach to mitigate potential bacterial decomposition of the dermis and/or epidermis in the diffusion cell across the study duration. The stability of drug in the receptor solution samples should be validated as part of the receptor sample analytical method validation.

Receptor Solution Sampling Qualification: The accuracy and precision of receptor solution sample collection at each time point should be appropriately qualified. For studies using a vertical diffusion cell, part of or the entire receptor solution volume should be removed and replaced at each time point to provide optimal solubility sink conditions. For studies using a flow-through diffusion cell, it is necessary to qualify the lengths of tubing and associated dead volumes and flow rate, to accurately calculate the lag time before a sample elutes through the tubing and is collected.

Receptor Solution Sample Analytical Method Validation: The receptor sample analysis procedures should be validated in a manner compatible with the current FDA Guidance for Industry on Bioanalytical Method Validation. The validation of the receptor sample analytical method should include relevant qualifications of dilution integrity as well as stability assessments with the highest relevant temperature in the receptor solution, which may be warmer than 32°C for the duration of the IVPT study (e.g., 34°C for 48 hours), or for the longest interval between sampling time points for methods in which the entire receptor solution is replaced at each sampling time point. If the samples are processed in specific ways for analysis (e.g., by drying and reconstituting the receptor samples in a smaller volume to concentrate the sample and increase the effective analytical sensitivity, or by dilution of receptor solution samples into the validated curve range of the analytical method) those procedures should be validated (e.g., by qualifying the dilution integrity during the analytical method validation). The stability of the drug in the receptor solution sample should be validated in a receptor solution matrix that has been exposed to the underside of the skin in a diffusion cell under conditions relevant to the pivotal study. A pre-dose "zero" sample should be collected from each diffusion cell in both the pilot and pivotal studies, as it may help to identify potential contamination associated with each skin section and/or each diffusion cell.

Environmental Control: Ambient laboratory temperature and humidity during the study should be monitored and reported. An environmentally controlled temperature range of 21°C ± 2°C and a humidity range of 50% ± 20% relative humidity are recommended.

Pilot Study: Following the method development studies, a pilot study with at least three skin donors and a minimum of four replicate skin sections should be performed on the formulations (including at least one control formulation to demonstrate method sensitivity, for example, at 50% of drug strength of one of the formulations being investigated) to be tested in order to estimate the number of donors required to power the pivotal study. In order to calculate statistical power, it is recommended that the arithmetic mean for each donor be determined and used as point estimates for each donor. Power analysis should then be performed using these point estimates as values.

Permeation Profile and Range: The flux profile and cumulative permeation profile of the drug across the range of sampling times, which corresponds to the study duration, should be characterised based upon the results of the pilot study. The pilot study results should be plotted with error bars, comparing the permeation profiles for the formulations in the pilot study, as separate plots for average pseudo steady-state flux and average cumulative permeation (see below). The results of the pilot study should validate that the study duration (range) is sufficient to characterise the cutaneous pharmacokinetics of the drug(s), including a sufficiently complete flux profile to identify the maximum (peak) flux and a decline in the flux thereafter across multiple subsequent time points. The results of the pilot study should also validate that the sampling frequency provides suitable resolution for the flux profile.

Precision and Reproducibility: The pilot study flux and cumulative permeation results should be tabulated for each diffusion cell and time point, with summary statistics to describe the intra-donor average, standard deviation, and %CV among replicates, as well as the inter-donor average, standard error, and %CV.

Recovery, Mass Balance, and Dose Depletion: The recovery of the permeated drug in the receptor solution may be characterised in each diffusion cell as the cumulative total permeation of drug in the receptor solution over the study duration. This may be expressed as a percentage of the amount of drug in the applied dose. The minimum amount of dose depletion (not accounting for skin content) may thereby be estimated and should be reported.

Discrimination or Sensitivity: The discrimination ability of the method is perhaps best described as the ability of the method to detect changes in the cutaneous pharmacokinetics of the drug as a function of differences in delivery. The method development study with, for example, different dose amounts (as described above) provides supportive evidence that the methodology is sensitive to differences in drug delivery.

Robustness: A primary assumption related to robustness testing is that the methodology developed performs consistently when all variables (e.g., temperature, stirring rate) are at optimum settings. A value of robustness testing is that it can verify whether the method continues to provide a consistent output when such variables are slightly varied, thereby qualifying operational ranges for those variables. However, the variability inherent in the permeability of human skin, may not allow such consistency, and as such, study procedures should be controlled as precisely as possible.

Pivotal Study and Data Presentation

After completion of the above, the appropriate protocol will have been developed and validated, and as such, the appropriate data generated. For each formulation tested, the flux (rate of drug permeation) should be plotted as J on the Y-axis in units of mass/area/time (e.g., $ng/cm^2/hr$) versus time on the X-axis. Such profiles commonly resemble plasma pharmacokinetic profiles, although flux is a rate, rather than a concentration. The extent of drug permeation should also be plotted as the cumulative amount of drug permeated on the Y-axis in units of mass/area (e.g., ng/cm^2) versus time on the X-axis. The maximum flux (J_{max}) at the peak of the drug flux profile should be calculated and this is analogous to a C_{max}. Similarly, the cumulative total permeation of drug across the study duration should be plotted and compared and this corresponds to the AUC of the incremental drug permeation profile. For statistical analysis, log transformed data should be used. A point estimate for each donor should be determined as in the pilot study, and these values tested in a statistically appropriate way (ANOVA, Tukey's HSD, etc.).

6.4 ACTIVITY/DISEASE MODELS

The major limitation of any permeation model is that it shows how the drug is moving into and through the biological tissue, but does not show how the formulation affects the skin and whether the drug is bio-available, engages the target, and is able to act on the desired pathway(s).

Testing of cosmetic and pharmaceutical excipients and active ingredients for possible irritation effects has seen a slow evolution since its inception in the early 1900s. In 1944, the first U.S. Food and Drug Administration-recognised animal testing was implemented. Known as the "Draize test" (from toxicologist Dr John Henry Draize), it utilised rabbits for ocular and skin irritation of cosmetics and personal care items. While advances in animal testing allowed a decrease from six test subjects to one to three rabbits per test, animal rights activists and government legislation continues to denounce the practice of animal testing for topical and transdermal medicines. Although the 7th amendment to the European Union Cosmetics Directive now forbids animal testing of cosmetics in Europe, irritation testing in up to two animal species (rodent and mini-pig) is still required by regulatory authorities for various toxicological studies prior to a new topical medicine approval (e.g., New Drug Application). In addition, the time and cost associated with failure in the clinic mean that there remains a range of *in vivo* animal models using fish, rodents, minipigs, and non-human primates that have been developed to mimic human skin diseases such as skin cancers (melanoma, Basal Cell Carcinoma, and Squamous Cell Carcinoma), atopic dermatitis, psoriasis, skin infections (acne, MRSA, viral infections, tinea pedea, etc.), alopecia, and wounds. Many models exploit genetic engineering, as many involve gene mutations. However, the increasing regulatory restrictions and ethical concerns around the use of these animals in product development (in much the same way as for cosmetics), with proponents arguing for its discontinuation because of the dissimilarities between animals and humans (including skin thickness, density, and immune system irregularities), has meant that over recent years, an array of RHE and human *ex vivo* skin activity and disease models have been developed, some of which are described below.

6.4.1 Reconstituted Human Epithelium Activity/Disease Models

From the 1980s, early RHE skin models originally allowed the differentiation of an intact stratum corneum at an air–liquid interface, and have now evolved to include collagen, fibroblasts, and melanocytes. Commercially available examples include EPISKIN (L'Oreal), EpiDerm (MatTek Corporation), and ZenSkin (ZenBio), and they have rapidly gained acceptability in topical product testing for various aspects of pharmacotoxicological and dermal irritation studies whilst contributing to the refinement, reduction, and replacement of whole animal testing. For example, irritation validated testing with standardised test materials using cell viability and the release of biomarkers has shown good correlation for corrosion and irritant effects with those observed *in vivo*.

RHE cultures obtained by culturing adult human keratinocytes on a collagen substrate (e.g., EpiDerm®, ZenSkin) permits terminal differentiation and the reconstruction of an epidermis with a functional horny layer. The general structure, composition, and aspects of biochemistry bear a close resemblance to human skin. Cell viability and release of biomarkers can be quantified as an indication of corrosive/irritant effects on the skin. The primary advantage of this model, in comparison to *ex vivo* human skin, is that it is highly reproducible and allows comparisons with formulations of known irritancy. The biggest limitation of commercially available RHE models is the relatively weak barrier function compared to human skin which can lead to false positives in toxicity studies; however, their relatively high sensitivity and weaker barrier function could be useful in terms of giving a worst case scenario result for a formulation. Additionally, this model allows ranking of formulations and actives compared to known irritants.

Most RHE models attempt to replicate "healthy" human skin, but adaptation to replicate skin disease in a controlled, reproducible, and qualifiable manner has become an increasing requirement in topical product development. Such skin disease models are generally developed in-house with the objective of screening drug candidates and/or formulations, but commercially available RHEs models are becoming available. For example, RHE models for inflammatory and autoimmune diseases have been developed, including for psoriasis and atopic dermatitis where the specific pathway leading to expression of the disease state is induced by a cytokine stimulation/inflammatory cocktail or by downregulation of filaggrin. Alternatively, a commercially available psoriasis RHE is available (for example MatTek), produced from normal human epidermal keratinocytes and psoriatic fibroblasts harvested from psoriatic lesions to form a multi-layered, differentiated tissue. The psoriasis tissues maintain a psoriatic phenotype, as evidenced by increased basal cell proliferation, expression of psoriasis-specific markers, and elevated release of psoriasis-specific cytokines. Morphologically, the tissue model reportedly closely parallels lesional psoriatic human tissues, but lacks the inflammatory cellular components. Skin-cancer models have been constructed by incorporating various tumour entities within the three-dimensional RHE matrix. The Melanoma model (again from MatTek) consists of human malignant melanoma cells (A375), normal, human-derived epidermal keratinocytes (NHEK) and normal, human-derived dermal fibroblasts (NHDF) which have been cultured to form a multi-layered, differentiated epidermis with melanoma cells at various stages of CM malignancy. Structurally, the Melanoma model is reported to closely mimic the progression of melanoma *in vivo*.

6.4.2   *Ex Vivo* Human Skin Activity/Disease Models

As discussed previously for IVPT, the use of *ex vivo* human skin in developing disease models has numerous advantages over the use of animals, synthetic alternatives, and reconstructed tissue models that lack the full structure, appendages, and requisite cells. For example, in addition to the prominent keratinocytes that make up the human skin strata, immune cells play a major role in the pathophysiology of skin biology. Although it is accepted that, as with the other models, *ex vivo* human skin will lack cell migration from the circulatory and lymph system into the dermis, unlike the others, it contains resident immune cells. These typically include lymphocytes, dendritic cells, and Langerhans cells. Of these, the resident memory T cells (TRM) are known to be potent mediators against infection and autoimmune disease and in *ex vivo* human skin, it has been shown that such resident T cells secrete inflammatory cytokines. *Ex vivo* human skin can be cultured for up ca. two weeks, and a combination of stimulatory cytokines can result in the involvement of not only immune cells, but also the release of chemokines, antimicrobial peptides and keratinocyte differentiation biomarkers associated with clinical psoriasis which can be analysed by quantitative reverse transcription polymerase chain reaction (qRT-PCR). Research has shown similar success with other inflammatory skin diseases (e.g., acute [Th2 mediated] and chronic atopic dermatitis [Th1 mediated], vitiligo, and alopecia), along with wound healing, skin ageing, damage, and environmental stress, various skin infections (bacterial and fungal) and complex multi-mechanistic skin diseases, such as acne and infected dermatitis.

For example, modified zone of inhibition assays (TurChub®) (Figure 6.3) and infected skin *ex vivo* models have been developed in order to enhance and support topical formulation development. The modified zone of inhibition assays includes all the barrier functions associated with the human skin, but with the skin mounted employing a gasket designed to prevent lateral diffusion of the active formulation around the edges of the skin and with the organism growing under the skin layer (stratum corneum, epidermal sheet, or even dermatomed skin in an agar matrix). The modified zone of inhibition assays is generally used in the early stages of formulation development as a medium throughput screen; the test measures inhibition

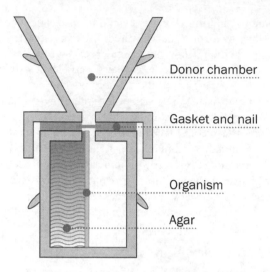

Donor chamber

Gasket and nail

Organism

Agar

FIGURE 6.3   Example zone of inhibition agar plate and MedPharm's TurChub® cell.

of organism growth (area of no growth) of the organism on the underlying agar. Furthermore, as the organism itself is used as the biomarker for permeation and anti-microbial activity, the test avoids the need for analytical methods (HPLC, UPLC, etc.) and multiple formulations containing different drugs can be screened at once, though "agar and drug compatibility" should be tested prior to starting the assay.

An advance on the relatively simple modified zone of inhibition assays are infected skin models. These rely on the ability to grow and culture the organisms on the skin, and to accurately recover and quantify the viable organisms after treatment. Typical organisms used (but not exclusively) are yeasts such as *C. albicans* or *P. ovale*, dermatophytes such as *T. rubrum* or *T. mentagrophytes*, or bacteria such as *P. acne*, *S. aureus* (including MRSA), *P. aeruginosa*, and *S. epidermis*. In these models, an organism (bacteria, yeast, or fungi) most relevant and causative of the infection is artificially introduced under controlled conditions and growth is controlled. The location of the infection within the skin is also controlled, for example, superficial or on the underside of the stratum corneum, epidermis, or dermis, such that the position of the organism within the skin closely resembles that of the clinical presentation. In addition, and if appropriate, the barrier properties of the diseased skin itself can be replicated. The ability of the drug or formulation to exert its anti-microbial effect is then assessed using the measurement of a biological marker in the form of ATP, a direct indicator of cell viability, PCR, or direct viable counts. This model also allows the use of living *ex vivo* skin to explore the effects of an infection and consequent inflammatory responses for multimodal mechanistic studies.

Both the infected skin models and the modified zone of inhibition assays are currently limited to mono-cultures, and thus only one organism is included in each replicate employed. However, advances in analytical techniques (e.g., differential PCR techniques), are leading to more complex biofilms (comprising multiple organism types in an infection) within the tissue to be explored. Furthermore, multifactorial diseases such as acne are also being advanced in order to combine the role of infection, inflammation and sebum production in the disease, allowing multiple outputs to be assessed and compared when evaluating drugs and/or formulations.

6.5 SUMMARY

As described above, there is a plethora of *in vitro* and *ex vivo* performance-testing models available to help topical and transdermal formulation development, and test conditions are rapidly advancing. IVRT provides a methodology to understand some thermodynamic mechanistic aspects of drug delivery, whilst also providing a means of assessing and comparing quality between products and during shelf-life thus reducing risk for the patient. IVPT provides an in vitro evaluation of drug delivery in the presence of skin itself and if performed with or in parallel with formulation assessment in the disease models (e.g., psoriasis, atopic dermatitis, bacterial infiltration, localised bacterial and fungal infections, and other dermatological indications), researchers can assess both drug delivery and target engagement (pharmacokinetics PKs and pharmacodynamics PDs) in a single assay from any formulation to assess PK/PD relationships. If such PK/PD models are not available, then some simplified models exist. For example, it is critical to understand the affinity of drugs to bind to different layers of tissue, because this can have a major impact on both penetration and potency. Thus skin-binding models have been developed that are similar to blood plasma-binding, but specific to skin proteins. If skin metabolism is a concern (see Chapter 1, Section 1.2.4) drug biotransformation can be assessed using several models such as keratinocytes, RHE, or a more holistic approach using freshly obtained human skin and monitoring metabolic pathway(s).

BIBLIOGRAPHY

Abd. E, Yousef, S.A., Pastore, N.A., Telaprolu, K., Mohammed, Y.H., Namjoshi, S., Grice, J.E., and Roberts, M.S. (2016). Skin models for the testing of transdermal drugs. *Clin. Pharm. Adv. Appl.* 8: 163–176.

Akhtar, S.A., Bennett, S.L., Waller, I.L., and Barry, B.W. (1984). An automated diffusion apparatus for studying skin penetration. *Int. J. Pharm.* 21: 17–26.

Ashtikar, M., Matthäus, C., Schmitt, M., Krafft, C., Fahr, A., and Popp, J. (2013). Non-invasive depth profile imaging of the stratum corneum using confocal Raman microscopy: first insights into the method. *Eur. J. Pharm. Sci.* 50: 601–608.

Bernard, G., Auger, M., Soucy, J., and Pouliot, R. (2007). Physical characterization of the stratum corneum of an in vitro psoriatic skin model by ATR-FTIR and Raman spectroscopies. *Biochim. Biophys. Acta* 1770: 1317–1323.

Bojar, R.A. (2015). Studying the human skin microbiome using 3D in vitro skin models. *Appl. In Vitro Toxicol.* 1: 165–171.

Bronaugh, R.L. (1998). Current issues in the *in vitro* measurement of percutaneous absorption. In: Roberts, M.S. and Walters, K.A. (Eds.), *Dermal Absorption and Toxicity Assessment*. New York, NY: Marcel Dekker, Inc., Chapter 5, pp. 155–159.

Bronaugh, R.L. and Stewart, R.F. (1985). Methods for in vitro percutaneous absorption studies IV: the flow-through diffusion cell. *J. Pharm. Sci.* 74: 64–67.

Bronaugh, R.L., Stewart, R.F., and Simon, M. (1986). Methods for in-vitro percutaneous absorption studies VII: use of excised human skin. *J. Pharm. Sci.* 75: 1094–1097.

Clowes, H.M., Scott, R.C., and Heylings, J.R. (1994). Skin absorption: flow-through or static diffusion cells. *Toxicol. In Vitro* 8(4): 827–830.

ECVAM (2009). *Performance Standards for In-Vitro Skin Irritation Test Methods Based on Reconstructed Human Epidermis.*

EMA (2014). *Concept Paper on the Development of a Guideline on Quality and Equivalence of Topical Products.* EMA/CHMP/QWP/558185/2014. London, UK: European Medicines Agency.

EURL ECVAM Scientific Advisory Committee (2016). *ESAC Opinion on the Validation Study of the epiCS® Skin Irritation Test (SIT) Based on the EURL ECVAM/OECD Performance Standards for In Vitro Skin Irritation Testing Using Reconstructed Human Epidermis (RhE).* ESAC Opinion No. 2016-05 of 24 June 2016; EUR 28177 EN. Luxembourg: Publications Office of the European Union.

European Food Safety Authority (2012). *Guidance on Dermal Absorption.* Luxembourg: Publications Office of the European Union.

EMA (2012). Guideline on quality of transdermal patches. In: *European Medicines Agency,* EMA/CHMP/QWP/911254/2011 2, Quality Working Party (QWP).

FDA (CDER) (1997). *Guidance for Industry – SUPAC-SS Non-Sterile Semisolid Dosage Form, Scale-Up and Post Approval Changes: Chemistry, Manufacturing and Controls; In Vitro Release Testing and In Vivo Bioequivalence Documentation.* Rockville, MD: U.S. Department of Health and Human Services.

FDA (2011). *FDA Draft Guidance Document on Cyclopirox which was revised in 2011.* Rockville, MD: U.S. Department of Health and Human Services

FDA (2016). *FDA Draft Guidance Document on Acyclovir Cream which was revised in 2016.* Rockville, MD: U.S. Department of Health and Human Services.

FDA (2017). *FDA Draft Guidance Document on Docosanol.* Rockville, MD: U.S. Department of Health and Human Services.

FDA (2017). *FDA Draft Guidance Document on Dapsone which was revised in 2017.* Rockville, MD: U.S. Department of Health and Human Services.

FDA (2016). *FDA Draft Guidance Document on Ivermectin.* Rockville, MD: U.S. Department of Health and Human Services.

FDA (2017). *FDA Draft Guidance Document on Silver Sulfadiazine.* Rockville, MD: U.S. Department of Health and Human Services.

FDA (2018). *FDA Guidance for Industry Bioanalytical Method Validation.* Rockville, MD: U.S. Department of Health and Human Services.

Franz, T.J. (1975). Percutaneous absorption on the relevance of in vitro data. *J. Invest. Dermatol.* 64: 190–195.

Franz, T.J. (1978). The finite dose technique as a valid in vitro model for the study of percutaneous absorption in man. *Curr. Probl. Dermatol.* 7: 58–68.

Franz, T.J., Lehman, P.A., and Raney, S.G. (2009). Use of excised human skin to assess the bioequivalence of topical products. *Skin Pharmacol. Physiol.* 22(5): 276–286.

Franzen, L., Selzer, D., Fluhr, J.W., Schaefer, U.F., and Windbergs, M. (2013). Towards drug quantification in human skin with confocal Raman microscopy. *Eur. J. Pharm. Biopharm.* 84: 437–444.

Guth, K., Schäfer-Korting, M., Fabian, E., Landsiedel, R., and Van Ravenzwaay, B. (2015). Suitability of skin integrity tests for dermal absorption studies in vitro. *Toxicol. In Vitro* 29: 113–123.

Haigh, J.M. and Smith, E.W. (1994). The selection and use of natural and synthetic membranes for in-vitro diffusion experiments. *Eur. J. Pharm. Sci.* 2(5–6): 311–330.

ICH (1995). Q2A: Text on validation of analytical procedures: definitions and terminology. *ICH Harmonised Tripartite Guideline.*

ICH (1996a). Q2B: Validation of analytical procedures: methodology. *ICH Harmonised Tripartite Guideline.*

ICH (1996b). Q2(R1): Validation of analytical procedures: methodology. *ICH Harmonised Tripartite Guideline.*

ICH (2003). Q1A(R2): Stability testing of new drug substances and products. *ICH Harmonised Tripartite Guideline.*

Kandárová, H., Liebsch, M., Genschow, E., Gerner, I., Traue, D., Slawik, B., and Spielmann, H. (2004). Optimisation of the EpiDerm test protocol for the upcoming ECVAM validation study on in vitro skin irritation tests. *ALTEX* 21: 107–114.

Kandárová, H., Liebsch, M., Gerner, I., Schmidt, E., Genschow, E., Traue, D., and Spielmann, H. (2005). EpiDerm skin irritation test protocol – assessment of the performance of the optimised test. *ATLA* 33: 351–367.

Kligman, A.M. and Christophers, E. (1963). Preparation of isolated sheets of human stratum corneum. *Arch. Dermatol.* 88(6): 702–705.

Küchler, S., Strüver, K, and Friess, W. (2013). Reconstructed skin models as emergingtools for drug absorption studies. *Expert Opin. Drug Metab. Toxicol.* 9(10): 1255–1263.

Lehman, P.A. and Franz, T.J. (2014). Assessing topical bioavailability and bioequivalence: a comparison of the in vitro permeation test and the vasoconstrictor assay. *Pharm. Res.* 31(12): 3529–3537.

Moghimi, H.R., Williams, A.C., and Barry, B.W. (1996a). A lamellar matrix model for stratum corneum intercellular lipids. I. Characterisation and comparison with stratum corneum intercellular structure. *Int. J. Pharm.* 131: 103–115.

Moghimi, H.R., Williams, A.C., and Barry, B.W. (1996b). A lamellar matrix model for stratum corneum intercellular lipids. II. Effect of geometry of the stratum corneum on permeation of model drugs 5-fluorouracil and oestradiol. *Int. J. Pharm.* 131: 117–129.

OECD (2004a). *428 European Commission Guidance Document on Dermal Absorption, Rev 7.* Paris: OECD Publishing.

OECD (2004b). *431 Guideline for the Testing of Chemicals. In Vitro Skin Corrosion: Reconstructed Human Epidermis (RhE) Test Method.* Paris: OECD Publishing.

OECD (2010). *439 Guideline for the Testing of Chemicals. In Vitro Skin Irritation: Reconstructed Human Epidermis Test Method.* Paris: OECD Publishing.

OECD (2015). *OECD Guideline for Testing of Chemicals, No. 439: In Vitro Skin Irritation: Reconstructed Human Epidermis Test Method.* Paris: OECD Publishing.

Organisation for Economic Co-operation and Development. (2011). *Guidance Notes on Dermal Absorption.* [Online] Available at: https://www.oecd.org/chemicalsafety/test ing/48532204.pdf [Accessed November 25, 2018].

Ph. Eur 1011, Patches, Transdermal, 01/2008:1011.

Raney, S.G., Franz, T.J., Lehman, P.A., Lionberger, R., and Chen, M.L. (2015). Pharmacokinetics-based approaches for bioequivalence evaluation of topical dermatological drug products. *Clin. Pharmacokinet.* 54(11): 1095–1106.

Ruela, A.L.M., Perissinato, A.G., de Sousa Lino, M.E., Mudrik, P., and Pereira, G.R. (2016). Evaluation of skin absorption of drugs from topical and transdermal formulations. *Braz. J. Pharm. Sci.* 52: 527–544.

Schäfer-Korting, M., Bock, U., and Diembeck, W. (2008). The use of reconstructed human epidermis for skin absorption testing: results of the validation study. *Altern. Lab. Anim.* 36: 161–187.

Schmook, F.P., Meingassner, J.G., and Billich, A. (2001). Comparison of human skin or epidermis models with human and animal skin in in-vitro percutaneous absorption. *Int. J. Pharm.* 215: 51–56.

Schreiber, S., Mahmoud, A., and Vuia, A. (2005). Reconstructed epidermis versus human and animal skin in skin absorption studies. *Toxicol. In Vitro* 19: 813–822.

Shah, V. (1998). *Topical Dermatological Drug Product NDAs and ANDAs: In Vivo Bioavailability, Bioequivalence, In Vitro Release and Associated Studies.* Rockville, MD: US Dept of Health and Human Services, pp. 1–19.

Skelly, J.P., Shah, V.P., Maibach, H.I., Guy, R.H., Wester, R.C., Flynn, G., and Yacobi, A. (1987). FDA and AAPS report of the workshop on principles and practices of in vitro percutaneous penetration studies: relevance to bioavailability and bioequivalence. *Pharm. Res.* 4: 265–267.

Todo, H. (2017). Transdermal permeation of drugs in various animal species. *Pharmaceutics* 9: 33–44.

Ueda, C.T., Shah, V.P., Derdzinski, K., Ewing, G., Flynn, G., Maibach, H., Marques, M., Rytting, H., Shaw, S., Thakker, K., and Yacobi A. (2009). Topical and transdermal drug products *Pharmacopeial Forum.* 35(4):750–764.

U.S. Food and Drug Administration (1997). *Guidance for Industry: Nonsterile Semisolid Dosage Forms Scale-Up and Postapproval Changes (SUPAC) – Chemistry, Manufacturing, and Controls: In Vitro Release Testing and In Vivo Bioequivalence Documentation.* Rockville, MD: FDA.

USP 40 General Information <1724> Semisolid products-performance testing.

Walters, K.A., Watkinson, A.C., and Brain, K.R. (1998). In vitro skin permeation evaluation: the only realistic option. *Int. J. Cosmet. Sci.* 20: 307–316.

Williams A.C., Cornwell P.A., and Barry B.W. (1992). On the non-Gaussian distribution of human skin permeabilities. *Int. J. Pharm.* 86: 69–77.

7 Process Development Considerations for Topical and Transdermal Formulations

7.1 INTRODUCTION

During the early stages of topical or transdermal drug development, generic methods of manufacture tend to be employed, taking account of the more obvious attributes of the compositional materials, and with observations being made of the processing parameters deployed. Once a lead formulation has been identified, or as it is sometimes called "locked", a phase of process development will be undertaken to identify potential causal relationships between the detailed specifications of component materials, the finer detail of processing parameters, and the quality attributes of the finished product. The aim is to produce batches that can be subsequently manufactured consistently and predictably and which possess the quality attributes which are critical to achieving the Target Product Profile.

The three principal attributes which can have a direct impact on the performance of all topical and transdermal products are the qualitative composition, the quantitative composition, and the physical microstructure. Performance in this context refers to both drug delivery (manifesting as therapeutic efficacy or indeed toxicity) and technical functionality, for example, flow properties, texture, spreadability, and adhesion. The manufacturing process can have a marked effect on the microstructure of the resultant finished product and can exert significant influence over product performance. Safety and efficacy are clearly of paramount importance in both clinical and regulatory contexts, but attributes such as appearance, texture, and spreadability for topical products and adhesivity for transdermal products can have a significant impact on patient acceptability, adherence, and as a consequence, commercial success – hence the importance of the manufacturing process.

When developing a manufacturing process for topical or transdermal drug products, it is always important to consider the impact of an ultimate change in production scale as the programme progresses towards commercialisation. The processes considered during the process development phase should be as representative as possible of a potential commercial-scale manufacture and should be designed such that the resulting formulation meets the critical quality attributes defined and laid down in the Target Product Profile and release specifications. Communication between formulation development groups and manufacturing groups is vital in ensuring similar equipment and previous data is used to enable smooth transfer of activities. Quality by Design (QbD), as introduced in Chapter 5, should be at the forefront of process development considerations, constantly linking process back to the Quality Target Product Profile (QTPP) and subsequent Critical Quality Attributes (CQAs).

Within this chapter, the basic principles of the manufacture of semi-solids (for example, ointments, creams, and gels) and transdermal patches are initially outlined, followed by an in-depth discussion of process development and scale-up considerations for topical semi-solids. Transfer of developed methods towards commercial scale manufacturer and process validation will also be discussed, including the importance of SUPAC when assessing formulation performance. Finally, a case study highlighting the importance of process development is included.

7.2   BASIC PRINCIPLES OF THE MANUFACTURE OF SEMI-SOLIDS AND TRANSDERMAL PATCHES

It should be noted that every formulation is unique and therefore, whilst generic manufacturing methods can be often used in the first instance, they will likely require optimisation, especially for scale-up.

7.2.1   Ointments

Ointments can either be prepared by incorporation or fusion techniques, depending on the active pharmaceutical ingredient(s) and the type of base used:

- Ointments containing hydrocarbon bases can be prepared by both techniques
- Ointments made using absorption bases tend to be prepared by fusion techniques, although levigation can be employed to assist wetting of solids
- Ointments formulated with emulsifying bases are prepared by fusion followed by mechanical addition
- Ointments made with water-miscible bases are prepared by fusion or incorporation depending on the solubility of the components of the formulation

The advantage of the incorporation method is that it avoids the use of heat, thereby making it a suitable manufacturing process for formulations containing thermolabile materials. Where the drugs or other solid components are insoluble in the ointment base, fusion methods are followed. These involve heating the components to a temperature higher than the melting point of all of the excipients and then cooling with mixing. It is this cooling step which will have the marked impact on the resulting formulation; simplistically, the faster the cooling rate, the more viscous the resultant formulation tends to be, and vice versa. In the manufacture of topical semi-solids, fusion techniques are more widely used in industry compared to that of incorporation.

7.2.2   Creams

A cream is a semi-solid emulsion containing a high proportion of water. The emulsion can be water-in-oil (w/o) where droplets of an aqueous phase (dispersed phase) are dispersed in oil (continuous phase), or oil in water (o/w) where the oil is the dispersed phase in an aqueous continuous phase. The following generic procedure is often used for the manufacture of cream formulations:

1. Separate vessels containing the oil and aqueous phases are prepared. Emulsifying agents can be added to either phase, depending on their hydro-philic-lipophilic balance (HLB), i.e., whether they are hydrophilic (water soluble) or hydrophobic (oil soluble).
2. The oil phase is heated to melt the solid components (where required) – usu-ally a few degrees above the highest melting point. The aqueous phase is also heated to the same temperature to avoid formation of a granular prod-uct through heterogeneous solidification when a hot oil phase is combined with a cool aqueous phase.
3. The dispersed phase is then added to the continuous phase and mixed using a suitable emulsification agitator while maintaining the temperature of the system. In general, and depending on the formulation composition, for emulsification to occur and result in a stable formulation, agitation should be high energy, such as that provided by a high-shear homogeniser. The energy supplied through a combination of high shear and mixing duration will produce uniform distribution of the desired droplet size (as further discussed below).
4. The mixture is then cooled to ambient temperature (or to product storage temperature) with constant mixing. It is possible to incorporate volatile and/ or heat-sensitive components during cooling stage.

Of the above processing parameters, it is the heating and cooling rates, and the agitation energy which tend to define the characteristics of the resulting product. Manufacturing scale, vessel dimensions and configuration, heating and cooling mechanisms, applied shear, screen type, and duration of homogenisation are there-fore important considerations. The manufacture of creams is a complex task and matching the exact procedure used under laboratory conditions can be challenging. Emulsification equipment can introduce energy into the system in different ways depending on the settings employed and the scale of manufacture. The choice of emulsification equipment depends on:

- Quantity of cream to be prepared
- Type of emulsifier/surfactant used
- Range of droplet size required
- The flow properties of the emulsion during the emulsification and cooling processes

The process employed, in addition to the choice of emulsifier, can directly affect the droplet size and ultimately the physical stability of the cream. Large droplets tend to cream and coalesce and a broad range in size distribution can encourage Ostwald ripening (described later). The most physically stable creams are there-fore those with small droplets (typically 0.2–10 μm) and a narrow size distribution.

The various categories of cream physical instability are shown diagrammatically in Figure 7.1 and are:

- *Creaming*: Where the dispersed droplets separate under the influence of gravity and occurs with large droplets. Most oil phases are lighter than water and therefore rise to the surface to form an upper layer of cream.
- *Flocculation*: A weak, reversible association between emulsion droplets which are separated by trapped continuous phase. Each cluster behaves as a single kinetic unit.
- *Coalescence*: An irreversible process where, in each dispersed phase, droplets merge together to form larger droplets until the cream cracks (or breaks) leading to complete separation of water and oil phases.
- *Ostwald ripening*: An irreversible process where larger droplets grow at the expense of smaller droplets. The more soluble smaller droplets dissolve and diffuse through the continuous phase and redeposit onto the larger droplets, which increase in size.
- *Phase inversion*: Occasionally occurs under specific conditions, for example, with changes in emulsifier solubility at different temperatures or through the interaction of other additives such as salts.

7.2.3 Gels

The manufacturing process for gels is largely dependent on the type of polymer used. For example, cellulose-based polymers tend to be dispersed or dissolved in a pre-heated portion of the water, or the organic phase (for example, propylene glycol or polyethylene glycol) before the remainder of the formulation (cold) is added. Similarly, carbomers are usually pre-dispersed in water and then the remainder of the formulation is added. Neutralisation of the carboxyl groups completes the hydration of the polymer. In all cases, it is recommended to review the guidelines from the polymer manufacturer, although most of these assume the use of simple aqueous solutions. Since the preferred log P of most drugs for skin permeation is <3.5, then low or non-aqueous formulations may be required, and this may well heavily influence the selection of gelling agent and commensurate process.

7.2.4 Transdermal Patches

The simplest and most common transdermal patch design is the drug-in-adhesive patch, formed using the following generic procedure:

1. Dissolve or disperse the drug (and polymer, plasticisers, where applicable) in the relevant adhesive. This also may include additional volatile processing solvents to aid manufacture.
2. In general, the adhesive mixture will then be coated to a defined thickness onto a release liner (or the backing layer), and the adhesive cured at predefined conditions of temperature and duration, depending on the type of adhesive used and the formulation composition.

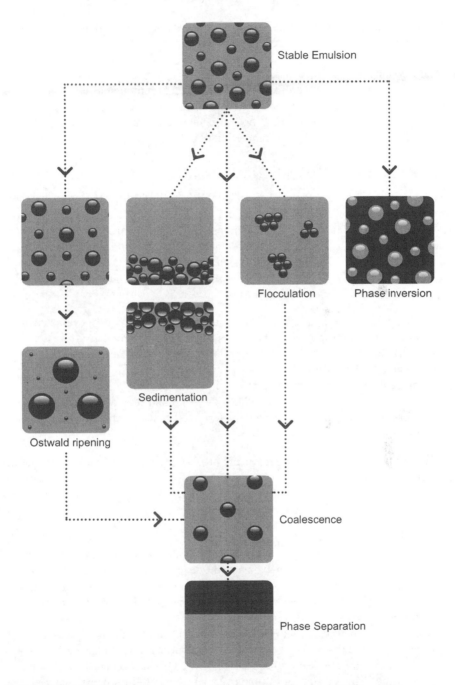

FIGURE 7.1 Schematic representation of instability mechanisms in the emulsion system. (Adapted from Hu, Y.T., Ting, Y., Hu, J.Y., and Hsieh, S.C., 2017. Techniques and methods to study functional characteristics of emulsion systems. *J. Food Drug Anal.* 25: 16–26.)

3. The backing layer (or release liner) is then applied before punching out of patches of the required size and packaging.

The coating and lamination steps are the most critical in order to produce a wrinkle-free laminate with uniform drug content and reproducible adhesive-coating thickness. To this end, the tensions used must be carefully controlled. Curing of the adhesive should also be monitored (both time and temperature) to avoid the formation of air bubbles and to ensure completion of curing.

7.3 PROCESS DEVELOPMENT AND SCALE-UP

The aim of process development is to establish optimal process parameters/conditions to manufacture the pharmaceutical product to meet quality and regulatory standards. Process development also demonstrates that the manufacturer of the pharmaceutical product has sufficient understanding of the manufacturing method, and has controls in place which are appropriate to maintain the quality of the product within the set quality specifications when scaled up. At the end of process development, the following questions should to be answered:

- Have the Critical Processing Parameters (CPPs) been fully evaluated to understand their impact on the CQAs of the finished product?
- What influence do the Critical Material Attributes (CMAs) have on the CPP and CQA? For example, how does changing the viscosity, particle size, or grade of one of the excipients affect the mixing time?
- What does the Design Space (DS) look like and how achievable is it to work within it, technically and in terms of cost (i.e., how robust is the process)?

Process risk assessment, manufacturing process, stability, and packaging and filling are discussed in further detail below. Since the acronyms CMA, CQA, and CPP are used extensively throughout this chapter, and in the discussion regarding process development, to assist the reader, they are defined as:

A **CMA** is "a physical, chemical, biological, or microbiological property or characteristic of an input material that should be within an appropriate limit, range, or distribution to ensure the desired quality of output material" (Maguire and Peng, 2015). An input material can include both the excipients and the API that make up the formulation and also include processing solvents like the volatile excipients.

A **CQA** is "a physical, chemical, biological, or microbiological property or characteristic that should be within an appropriate limit, range, or distribution to ensure the desired product quality. CQAs are generally associated with the drug substance, excipients, intermediates (in-process materials), and drug product" (Maguire and Peng, 2015).

A **CPP** is "a process parameter whose variability has an impact on a CQA and therefore should be monitored or controlled to ensure the process produces the desired quality" (EMA, 2001).

7.3.1 PROCESS RISK ASSESSMENT

The concept of risk assessments was introduced in Chapter 5, and they are typically rolling documents where the impact of any identified risk is re-assessed throughout the development pathway. The document should be produced prior to initiating any experimental process development. At the start, the risks will be generic, but as knowledge is acquired then the risks and mitigation strategy will become defined and refined. To identify the risks associated with the manufacturing process, the following need to be understood:

1. The finished product CQAs, for example, dissolution time, content uniformity, process impurities, IVRT.
2. Formulation composition and the likely CMAs, for example, the polydispersity of a polymer, viscosity grades, hydration time, heat stability.
3. The basic processes required in manufacturing and their likely impact on the product's CQAs; examples of CPPs include the order of addition, processing temperature, mixing speeds, holding times, homogeniser opening diameters or shapes.

Some of the risk assessment procedures that can be used are: Failure Mode Effects Analysis (FMEA); Failure Mode, Effects and Criticality Analysis (FMECA); Fault Tree Analysis (FTA); Hazard Analysis and Critical Control Points (HACCP); Hazard Operability Analysis (HAZOP); Preliminary Hazard Analysis (PHA); and risk ranking and filtering. The approach adopted will be based partly on the prior experience of the manufacturing organisation and partly on the complexity of the manufacturing process.

The following should be evaluated during process risk assessments:

1. *Risk identification*: What might go wrong in the case of manufacturing process. This is usually linked to a negative impact on the CQA (failure mode). For example, a potential failure could be inadequate mixing of the formulation, resulting in a heterogeneous product.
2. *Risk analysis*: Qualitative and quantitative measurement of the probability of occurrence, the potential severity of the outcome, and in some cases, the detectability of the failure mode. Each criterion will be ranked (typically from 1–5, although it is common for severity to have a higher degree of weighting depending on the assessment) and the product of these elements gives a numerical value (risk score) to the relevant risk. For example, in an FMEA, this score is referred to as the risk priority number (RPN).
3. *Risk evaluation*: Is the level of risk deemed to be acceptable or is immediate action required? For example, if the RPN is above a certain pre-defined level, strategies for risk mitigation are required. Certain failure modes would therefore be classified as high, medium, and low risk.
4. *Risk control*: This includes risk reduction (the process of reducing the risk to an acceptable level) and risk acceptance.
5. *Risk communication*: Sharing of information.

To aid the risk assessment process the following can be used:

Process flowchart: A good flowchart should map the manufacturing process and will help understanding of the process to identify potential failure modes. The flowchart should indicate the material flow, processes, in-process checks and various processing stage gates.

IPO: An input (I), process (P), output (O) assessment can be performed to aid the FMEA risk assessment. It is important to have an initial understanding of the manufacturing process such that the IPO can be defined. For example, in the manufacture of creams, there are multiple steps one of which may be: *Input*: Oil phase excipients; *Process*: Heating; *Output*: Clear melt obtained. The potential failure mode for this would therefore be insufficient heating/melting of the oil phase excipients, which could impact the homogeneity of the formulation.

It is not just the process that needs to be considered during the risk assessment, but also the input materials. Each input material will have a corresponding specification, which may or may not impact on the final product quality. It is appropriate to lock the material specifications before proceeding to process development. The majority of excipient suppliers will support product development by providing samples that extend across the specification ranges (where possible); such samples are typically known as QbD samples. Ideally, knowledge of the CMAs and their impact on the CQA of the product should be assessed as early as possible in the development process to mitigate the risk of multiple, and potentially expensive, changes further down the line. However, as previously described, some CMAs may only be identified at the process development stage (for example, excipient viscosity and mixing time).

The product risk assessment process is used to identify the CQAs and the CPPs. Most of the CQAs are eventually listed on the product release and shelf-life specification and their limits established during process development. Some potential CQAs include (but are not limited to):

- *Drug product appearance*: Changes in appearance of a product could indicate chemical or physical instability. For example, a cream may show non-uniform phase distribution which could indicate potential phase separation of the dispersed and continuous phase. Appearance can be affected by aeration, droplet size, presence of degradation products (of drug or excipients), or process contamination.
- *Microscopic appearance*: Changes in the microstructure could indicate a potential physical stability problem, for example, a change in droplet size.
- *pH/apparent pH*: Changes in pH may affect physical, chemical, or microbial stability of the drug product during or following processing.
- *Apparent viscosity*: Viscosity can affect usability (e.g., dosing from a tube) and can have an impact on drug release from the formulation to the site of action.
- *Drug assay*: Any impact on the percentage label claim of the product could be indicative of degradative processes or drug:excipient binding.

- *Drug-related substances*: Depending on the degradation pathway of the drug substance in the formulation, some processes may have a detrimental effect on the stability of the drug, leading to an increase in the level of drug-related substances. The processes should be selected to minimise this risk.
- *Content uniformity*: In order that a safe and effective dose is administered, it is important that the manufacturing processes achieve uniformity in distribution of the drug throughout the manufactured batch.
- *Antioxidant/preservative assay (where applicable)*: Similarly to the drug assay, the processes used should not affect the assay of other key or essential ingredients.
- *In vitro* performance of the drug product, including drug release/dissolution and drug skin permeation testing: The manufacturing process can impact the microstructure and rheological profile of semi-solid drug products, which can impact *in vitro* performance test data.

When developing a manufacturing process, any of the above or their derivative responses can be considered as an output.

7.3.2 MANUFACTURING PROCESS

In order to reproducibly manufacture a pharmaceutical product, a set of established and validated processes are required (process validation is discussed in more detail in Section 7.4.2). Examples of processes used to prepare topical formulations include emulsification, gelation, hydration, and dissolution. Each of these should be designed with consideration of the physicochemical properties of the API/excipient, such as its degradation pathways, solubility, and melting point. For example, the droplet size in an emulsion will depend on the type of surfactant, the charge, HLB values, and homogeniser head design, et cetera.

7.3.2.1 Manufacturing Equipment Considerations

7.3.2.1.1 Process and Equipment Selection

As outlined above, each type of topical or transdermal product will involve different processes and therefore different types of equipment. Some of the processes commonly used are listed in Table 7.1.

As shown, process selection and equipment are linked to the desired output. For example, the viscosity of the solution will dictate the type of paddles and motor power to be used.

7.3.2.1.2 Manufacturing Equipment Capacity

Most manufacturing equipment is designed to give the optimum product output when used within their operational ranges. Equipment optimum capacity is identified during installation. For example, a 12–15 L vessel would be an appropriate size to manufacture a 10 kg batch. However, using a 100 L vessel for a 10 kg batch size is likely to lead to poor product consistency due to improper product flow caused by partially submerged mixing blades. Similarly, mixing paddles should be the correct dimensions to ensure full agitation of the whole batch of product, otherwise the

TABLE 7.1
Ideal Processes Used in Topical Manufacturing and the Expected Output

Processes	Examples of Expected Output of the Process
Mixing	A homogenous mixture/solution
Homogenising	A bi-phasic system with a dispersed phase uniformly distributed in a continuous phase
	Droplet size reduction
Heating	Changing the state of matter from solid to liquid or semi-solid to assist flow, handling, and processing during manufacturing
Cooling	Changing the state of matter from liquid to solid or semi-solid to provide structure to the formed product
	Cooling to allow handling

resulting formulation may not be homogenous, impacting drug content uniformity, visual appearance, pH, and viscosity.

7.3.2.1.3 Equipment Energy Requirements

Similar to the capacity of the equipment used, the energy required for each process will depend on the batch size and the physical properties of the end/intermediate product. For example, during the manufacturing process for polymer hydration, the mixing equipment and its power draw need to be considered in light of the resulting viscosity of the product.

Computational fluid dynamics (CFDs) and computational fluid mixing (CFM) can be used in conjunction with experimental data to establish optimum mixing methods. Essentially, the mixing process depends on the transition from laminar to turbulent flow within the body of material, via application of an inertial force. Working against this transition is the viscosity of the material. The Reynolds equation establishes the ratio of the inertial force against the viscous force, and this is known as the Reynolds number R_e:

$$R_e = \frac{\rho v L}{\mu} \tag{7.1}$$

where ρ is the fluid material density in Kg/m^3; v is the velocity of the fluid in m/s; L is the length or diameter of the flow surface in m; and μ is the viscosity of the fluid in Ns/m^2. If the Reynolds number is <2000, then flow is laminar, if 2000–4000, then flow is transitional, and if it is >4000, then flow will be turbulent.

Most semi-solid manufacturing methods involve a degree of high-shear processing. This may be in the form of direct homogenisation or may occur as a result of forced passage through orifices such as those which might be implicated in discharging the vessel, piping the material between processing equipment, or ejection during filling processes. The Power Law index can be used to evaluate the magnitude of shear thinning or thickening which might occur at such high-shear rates. Using data obtained from a shear rate ramp curve, the behaviour under high shear can be defined as shear thinning or thickening and the extent of this behaviour can be quantified. The power law region of the curve shows linearity on a log–log plot of viscosity vs. shear rate but exhibits power law dependence on a linear scale plot.

The Power Law (or Ostwald de Waele Model) can be used to mathematically express the power law region of a flow curve as follows:

$$\sigma = k\gamma^n: \text{ Power law index} \qquad (7.2)$$

or

$$\eta = k\gamma^{n-1}: \text{ Power law index} \qquad (7.3)$$

where:
  k = consistency
  η = viscosity
  n = power law index
  σ = shear rate
  γ = shear rate consistency

Such modelling can be used to predict optimal processing methods to achieve the required CQAs.

7.3.2.2   Process Dynamics Involved in Manufacturing Topical Formulations

Understanding each process for product manufacture will ultimately inform all scale-up operations from laboratory to a commercial manufacturing facility. Early investigations of process dynamics during the formulation development phase will save time and effort at a later stage.

7.3.2.2.1   Dissolution of the API

Where the drug substance is in solution within the drug product, a good understanding of its solubility and dissolution is fundamental to establishing the manufacturing process. API particle size and polymorphic form are examples of factors affecting drug dissolution. Dissolution rates may be enhanced through reduction in the particle size of any solid drug substance. Micronisation can be achieved through a number of different methods adapted to the scale of operation. Once optimised, any change in the particle size distribution (PSD) of the API will impact its dissolution rate, and hence it is important to maintain the PSD throughout the process development and scale-up stages. It is sometimes believed that where the drug is in solution within a formulation, polymorphic form should not be a consideration for process development. However, the presence of different polymorphs may alter the drug dissolution time, the heating required to get the same amount of the drug dissolved in the vehicle, and drug stability. Care should be taken to avoid the potential for the process to cause the drug to precipitate out, particularly where this may lead to new polymorphic forms which are less soluble and/or stable. A change in the polymorphic form of the API over time could result in a change in process time and

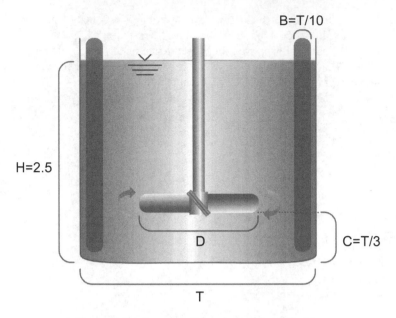

B=T/10

H=2.5

D

C=T/3

T

D = Diameter of mixing head (paddle)
B = Baffles
C = Off-bottom clearance
T = Tank diameter
H = Height of the fill volume

FIGURE 7.2   A typical mixing vessel.

or incomplete dissolution of the drug, resulting in a drug product which fails to meet its specification criteria. It is therefore advisable to monitor the polymorphic form used during process development and scale-up by performing x-ray diffractometry or thermal analysis.

7.3.2.2.2   Mixing/Blending Process

Mixing/blending are important processes because they transform a non-uniform mixture into one that is uniform. Parameters which should always be taken into consideration in the mixing/blending process, and particularly in scale-up, are the vessel geometry and the mixing mechanism. The vessel should be constructed using dimensions calculated in relation to the diameter of the vessel (Figure 7.2), and when scaling up, it is important to retain geometric similarity.

Use of the scalability constant allows further scaling to maintain the ratio of the vessel's dimensions. Most mixing is carried out using axial or radial type/mixers. Myers et al. (1996) compiled a list of some of the impeller types and their application. Different products have different viscosities for which different types of impellers are recommended. The ideal impeller type for different viscosities is illustrated in Figure 7.3.

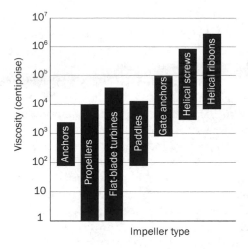

FIGURE 7.3 Impeller-type selection based on viscosity.

Flow dynamics/patterns of mixing are linked to impeller type and any baffle systems which might be in place to introduce turbulence in mixing. Baffle systems can only be implemented for low viscosity, free-moving fluids. In the event that the mixing time needs to be shortened, the turbulence in the system can be increased. An increase in the stirrer speed may not increase the turbulence significantly. Hence, baffles are introduced on the wall of the vessel, which introduce axial and radial flow patterns, increasing turbulence significantly. As previously discussed, the power of the motor should also be considered.

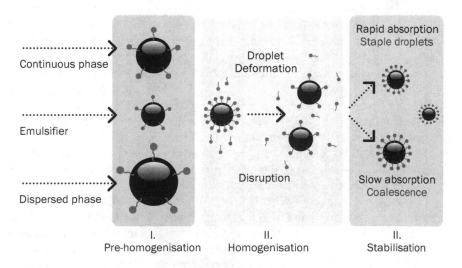

FIGURE 7.4 The process of droplet size reduction.

7.3.2.2.3 Optimisation of Droplet Size

As previously highlighted, for semi-solid emulsion formulations such as creams, the droplet size and uniformity of droplet distribution can be considered a CQA. Although droplet size can often be largely attributed to the surfactant used and its concentration, it is also dependent upon the viscosity ratio of the continuous phase to the dispersed phase and can be altered by the application of high shear in the manufacturing process. Homogenisers are often used to uniformly reduce the droplet size of and distribute the dispersed phase. As discussed in Section 7.2.2, small droplets (in the range 0.2 and 10 μm) are more likely to produce a stable emulsion and are therefore generally preferred.

Droplet size reduction occurs though the processes illustrated in Figure 7.4. Homogenisation can be achieved through ultrasonic disruption, high pressure, or mechanical means. The most common technique deployed in the processing of pharmaceutical semi-solids is mechanical high-shear rotor stator homogenisation. This reduces the droplet size by drawing the mixture upwards from the bottom of the vessel and transporting it through the radial opening of the rotor system. The mixture is horizontally forced outwards, at high velocity, through perforations in the work head screen. Such high shear and the turbulent flow that arises leads to the disruption of the droplets. A range of work heads and screens are available with difference size perforations to achieve the desired droplet size and distribution. When scaling a process, there is no single parameter that can be applied to high-shear rotor/stator mixers; rotor tip speed, work head design, power input, volume turnover, liquid rheology (characteristics of the liquid under shear), and viscosity all affect the end result.

7.3.2.2.4 Heating and Cooling Rate

For any process that involves fusion (for example, in the manufacture of ointments), the heating and cooling rates are important parameters affecting the final product. Solid components of the formulation require heating in order to melt before they are mixed with the liquid-based excipients. Slower heating rates result in a longer overall heating time which may lead to some loss of the most volatile components through evaporation. On the other hand, heating too rapidly may burn or degrade ingredients at the contact surface of the heat exchange; hence the heating rate should be carefully selected. Upon cooling of the mixture, the formulation starts to thicken as the excipient mixture start to solidify. Assuming that cooling is uncontrolled (i.e., the heat source is removed and the vessel is left at ambient temperature), the rate of cooling is greatest immediately following removal of the heat source because the temperature difference between the product and its environment is at its maximum. The rate of cooling then starts to plateau as a result of increase in viscosity. The formation of the formulation microstructure can be highly dependent upon cooling rate, which influences the product viscosity and rheological behaviour.

It is also important to consider the process of heat transfer when the formulation thickens. Generally, the formulation at the extremities of the bulk (i.e., close to the side of the vessel) will cool at a faster rate. Therefore, careful design of the paddles used during mixing is required. Often, anchor paddles are fitted with wall scrapers to prevent the build-up of cooled material between the paddle and the vessel wall.

7.3.2.2.5 Uniformity of Dosage Form

It is important to determine the uniformity of the manufactured formulation for quality, and ultimately for safety and efficacy reasons. This can be by assessing the drug and essential excipient content, apparent pH, viscosity, and/or appearance (macro- and microscopic) at different locations within the bulk, during the manufacturing process, and within the bulk and primary packaged product. It is important to note that multiple tests should be performed to avoid false positives. For example, once the drug is in solution, the drug content throughout the bulk is likely to be homogenous. However, the formulation may contain unhydrated polymer which may result in heterogeneous viscosity and particulates visually observed.

7.3.2.2.6 Polymer Hydration or Solvation

Hydration or solvation of the gelling agent is important for the formation of a gel and to build the viscosity of a solution. Different type of gelling agents will hydrate and gel differently. For example, carbomer hydration and gelation is pH dependent, but that of hypromellose (HPMC) and hydroxyl ethyl cellulose (HEC) is pH independent. Carbomers rely on their carboxyl group being activated (generally above pH 5) and then neutralised to form cross-links and gel.

7.3.2.3 Process Designing

Based on the understanding of the formulation and the processes involved during the manufacture, one can design the manufacturing process by defining the order of addition, the process steps, and the process timing, heating, and cooling rates.

7.3.2.3.1 Protection of API during Manufacturing

Understanding the degradation pathways of the drug substance within a formulation is critical to the design of the manufacturing process. Some APIs are known to be sensitive to light, temperature, oxygen, or moisture. For example, retinoic acid compounds are sensitive to both ultraviolet (UV) light and oxygen. These APIs can be protected by using appropriate light filters in the processing facility and by using closed system equipment with a blanket of nitrogen, argon, or another inert gas.

7.3.2.3.2 Order of Addition

Order of addition plays a key role in the formation of simple or complex formulations. Sometimes the order of addition can negatively influence the outcome of a formulation, for example, phase inversion in creams when particular surfactants are used. Ideally, the drug will be dissolved in the excipient in which it has the highest solubility, followed by the slow addition of excipients in which the drug is less soluble. The slow addition helps prevent precipitation of the drug out of solution.

Where excipients are solid, these will either be dissolved in a solvent or will be melted to allow mixing and homogenising. Where melting is necessary, the remaining excipients should also be heated to the same temperature prior to mixing to avoid formation of a granular product through too-rapid cooling and heterogeneous solidification.

Some gelling agents take time to hydrate and form the gel matrix. Successful hydration relies on the particle size of the polymer, the method and speed of addition, and the particle dispersion in the solvent system. Carefully controlled addition into the solvent system may be sufficient to achieve hydration, but a potential alternative method to avoid the formation of lumps during the addition of the gelling agent is to disperse into an antisolvent prior to addition into the hydrating solution. This practice is commonly used in industry to speed up the manufacturing time without impacting the quality of the product. For example, HPMC is insoluble in water at 70°C; however, it dissolves in water at room temperature. This property of HPMC has been utilised to reduce the hydration time. Alternatively, HPMC can be dispersed in an antisolvent which is already present in the formulation composition, for example, ethanol or isopropyl alcohol, thus reducing the dispersion time, preventing lump formation, and decreasing the hydration time as the particles are finely dispersed in the solution. Similar measures may be taken with other polymers, although it is always best practice to seek any specific manufacturer's guidelines for use, albeit that such process may not always be directly transferable, as every formulation is unique.

7.3.2.3.3   Processing Steps

Processing steps should be defined by the minimum number of steps required to achieve the product. Some common steps involved in the processing of common topical formulations and transdermal patches are:

Gel: Dissolution of API → mixing of other components → gelation of polymer → pH adjustment (if required)

Cream: Dissolution of API → mixing of other components → heating of different phase→ homogenisation → cooling whilst mixing

Ointments: Dissolution of API (although depending on ointment base, heating may be required to facilitate dissolution) → heating to melt the solid components → mixing → cooling

Transdermal patches: Dissolution of API → mixing of adhesive and remaining formulation components → coating on release/backing liner → heating/curing of the adhesive → application of the backing liner

At the end of each processing step, expected observations should be defined; for example, a clear solution following dissolution, visually homogenous mixture at the end of mixing, a high viscosity white cream at the end of cooling. Based on these definitions, the duration of each process (for example, the length of time for homogenisation, the rate of cooling) may be established and in-process controls/checks (IPCs) can be defined.

7.3.2.3.4   In-Process Checks (IPCs)

In-process checks are normally performed to ensure the process has not deviated from what is expected. For example, a content uniformity test at various locations in the bulk after the mixing process will help understand the uniformity of product. As IPCs are performed to ensure the quality of the product during manufacturing, most IPCs are a subset of the final product specification – for example, drug assay and related substances, pH, macroscopic and microscopic observations. A process flowchart is a handy tool along with a process risk assessment (Section 7.3.1) to assess and identify the IPC requirements.

7.3.2.4   Process Optimisation

7.3.2.4.1   Defining and CPPs and CQAs

Building on the CPPs listed in Chapter 5, commonly evaluated CPPs for topical formulations and transdermal formulations are provided below, with an explanation of why they are considered critical.

1. *Drug dissolution time*: Dissolution time is dependent upon the intrinsic solubility, the processing temperature, the energy applied through agitation, and the wetting of the API by the solvent. Changes to API particle size distribution or the API polymorph used will adversely impact dissolution and dissolution rate, hence the relationship between these parameters should be established early on and controlled appropriately. Topical and transdermal drug delivery is contingent, in the first instance, on presentation of the drug in solution, hence the dissolution step in the manufacturing process is of paramount importance. Care should be taken in establishing dissolution, since in some instances the presence of an insoluble impurity can falsely suggest incomplete drug solubilisation.

2. *Order of addition*: Order of addition has been discussed above. Although order of addition is defined during the process design stage, it is important to revisit the order of addition during process optimisation. For example, when manufacturing a cream with a protein as an active in the lab, the protein may be added directly to the aqueous phase before homogenisation; however, because of the longer duration of heating during the scale-up process, it may not be feasible to add the protein to the aqueous phase before homogenisation due to high shear and high temperature susceptibility of the protein. Hence, a portion of water along with the protein may be selected for later addition to the homogenised phase of the cream. Order of addition should be selected such that there are minimal changes to the microstructure of the formulation.

3. *Agitation parameters*: Mixing and homogenisation introduce energy in the form of mobility and shear. Mechanical shear can have a significant impact on the individual formulation components, on the microstructure of the finished product, and on its physical characteristics. Depending on the properties of the component materials, the formulation may be shear-thinning, shear-thickening, or Newtonian in behaviour. The relationship between agitation parameters and physical characteristics is particularly marked with emulsion systems, which can form spontaneously, but to produce a viable and stable pharmaceutical formulation, energy in the form of mechanical shear is usually required. Simple paddle mixers can be used to produce droplet sizes of around 10 μm, but higher shear achieved through mechanical, ultrasonic or high-pressure homogenisation can result in emulsions with an average droplet size as low as 0.2 μm. In general, smaller droplet sizes result in higher viscosity semi-solids. Rheological profiles (including viscosity) not only inform subsequent manufacturing steps such as filling, but they can also have a significant impact on the performance of the product in clinical use. The amount of energy introduced into the manufacturing process is ultimately dependent upon the mechanical power (e.g., mixer speed, homogeniser rpm,

homogenisation pressure) and the duration of the intervention; hence, mixer speeds and mixing times are typical examples of processing parameters investigated for criticality. Potential undesirable consequences of agitation processes include heat generation, aeration, and spills. Aeration can lead to formulation heterogeneity and instability, especially in emulsion systems. Some viscosity modifying agents and polymers are also known to be incompatible with the high shear that accompanies homogenisation (for example, carbomers). Also worthy of consideration is the fact that the physical agitation induced by mixing can in some cases lead to component loss; for example, if a volatile solvent is present, mixing rate, along with the heat applied and generated by the process can lead to evaporation. Mitigation against all of these undesirable effects is possible through a combination of engineering controls and optimisation and control of agitation processes.

4. *Heating*: As previously outlined, in order to achieve homogeneity of the final finished drug product, excipients with melting points above room temperature will be required to be heated to a liquid state during the manufacturing process; however, the application of heat may be detrimental to the stability of the excipient itself or that of other components including the drug substance, and as such the effect of the heating process should be investigated and controlled accordingly.

5. *Cooling rate*: Some formulations incorporate excipients which solidify at room temperature; others may include thickening or gelling agents. In either case, cooling rates can have a significant impact on the resultant microstructure and, by consequence, the performance of the formulation. The greater order resulting from faster cooling and the commensurate higher energies implicated in phase transition generally lead to a more ordered structure, higher viscosity, and greater stability, and importantly, these attributes can ultimately affect formulation performance.

6. *Hold time*: Each manufacturing process involves various stages. It is important to understand the duration of the time that each stage can be held before proceeding to the next stage of manufacturing without affecting the quality of the end product. The hold time for different manufacturing stages is achieved through hold time studies (see Section 7.3.3.1).

7. *Curing time and temperature in transdermal patch manufacture*: This would ultimately depend on the choice of adhesive and plasticiser and other polymers. However, careful consideration to the drug stability and characteristics of the patch should be taken.

8. *Heating rate and direction of heat in transdermal patch manufacture*: The direction of heat (for example, above or below the patch) can influence the introduction of air pockets in the adhesive layer resulting in a non-uniform product. Careful control of the rate of heating can also assist in reducing the likelihood of this occurring.

7.3.2.4.2   The Design Space and DoE

As introduced in Chapter 5, Design of Experiment (DoE) is a tool that can help reduce the number of experiments required to arrive at an optimal process parameter range. In process development, understanding the optimal process parameter ranges will help the formulator/process engineer to define the DS of the process. Previously, the practice to optimise process experiments would be to perform experiments by changing one factor at a time (OFAT). However, this requires multiple experiments to generate the optimal result. DoE efficiently reduces the number of experiments required to generate the optimal solution and also establishes if there are any factors that have synergistic effects. Selecting the right factors for a DoE to optimise the process is critical; hence, the selection of the CPP and the response (quality characteristics being measured at each run in the experiment) is very important. These must be numeric, and the values must be sensitive enough to reflect changes in the process or product as the run conditions are changing. The response needs to be accurately measurable and directly related to, or should have a well-established relationship to, the CQAs.

Typically, two to three CPPs, based on importance to the product, will be selected for process optimisation. Going above the three factors (CPPs) markedly increases the number of experiments, cost, and time of optimisation. For process optimisation, mostly factorial and response surface design may be used depending on the objective. If more than three factors are to be tested, then the formulator can use a low-resolution fractional factorial design to screen the factors affecting the process significantly. The selected factors can then be evaluated further by using a higher resolution factorial DoE. Based on the DoE studies, the optimal ranges for the CPPs may be defined. The process robustness can be further established by running an additional DoE. The design space can then be used during the scale-up process.

7.3.2.5 Process Confidence

Once the manufacturing parameters and design space are defined, it is advisable to run a scale-up technical batch in a Good Manufacturing Practice (GMP) setting to confirm the optimum manufacturing method from the process development experiments. This should be prior to any GMP clinical trial manufacture to determine whether any quality impacting parameters have been missed or if any further clarity is required for the clinical trial manufacture documentation records.

7.3.3 STABILITY STUDIES

As part of the process development and scale-up, it is important to monitor the stability of the product, both in terms of intermediate stages throughout the manufacture (hold time studies) and of the finished, filled product to ensure that there are no chemical or physical changes when increasing the scale of manufacture.

7.3.3.1 Hold Time Studies

Hold time studies are designed to understand the short-term stability of the product during the intermediate stages of manufacturing. Although continuous manufacturing processes are increasingly popular for high volume products, there are other products for which the process is susceptible to planned or unplanned interruption. In such cases, hold time studies should be carried out to confirm that these interruptions do not have a detrimental impact on the finished product quality. The output of this study would be a recommended maximum hold time for each intermediate stage. Once this data is established, it can be assured that the product will meet the specification and/ or the CQA, even after unforeseen delays in manufacturing the final product.

Hold time studies follow a similar pattern to ICH stability programmes, although the specification tests and ranges of acceptance may be tailored to ensure processability is maintained, for example, aspects of the rheological profile of an intermediate may be critical for the process and may change over time, for example, of thixotropic systems. The primary container used in hold time studies should be demonstrably similar to that in which the product would be stored in practice, should the need arise.

7.3.3.2   ICH Stability

The final product, manufactured using the optimised process should be evaluated for long-term ICH stability (ICH Q1A[R2]), as outlined in Chapter 5. The stability specification should take into account all CQAs.

7.3.4   FILLING AND PACKAGING CONSIDERATIONS

Various factors may influence the filling of semi-solid product into its primary container. Some of the factors that need to be considered during scale-up include the rheology of the product, the flow behaviour of the product when subjected to stress, and the physical stability and recovery of the product after being exposed to the filling stresses and pressures on a filling machine.

Primary packaging is required to pack the product in to a usable container closure system. As the primary packaging is in contact with the product, it is important to understand factors that may affect product quality. Some of the factors that need to be considered for the packaging process during scale-up are:

- The design of the container closure system and whether it is suitable for filling the product using existing machinery
- Packaging availability for continuous supply
- Confirming the quality of the container closure system (although this is best defined much earlier in the development pathway) and understanding the supplier's acceptable quality limits (AQLs)
- Storage conditions of the primary packaging
- Cleaning protocols for the packaging and filling equipment before and after filling
- Methods of ensuring seal integrity and the processes and IPC required to assure maintenance of CQAs and optimal process efficiency
- Labelling, both in terms of the art work quality and stability

7.3.5   SCALE-UP CONSIDERATIONS

Equipment capacity and energy requirements were previously discussed above and, in conjunction with process dynamics, form the basis for considerations of scale.

Batch size selection: Although exceptions are not uncommon, a widely accepted rule of thumb in scale-up is that a multiplication factor of 10 can be used without undue risk when scaling a process (EMA, 2001). This multiple of 10 makes for easier scale-up calculations and identification of potential errors. For example, the process employed for a 1 kg batch can be employed for a 10 kg batch, but not for a 100 kg. The multiplication factor applied must be justified, and derivation through formal risk assessment is recommended – multiplication factors as low as 3 or 4 are often necessary to give the appropriate level of quality assurance for more complex processes. The factor also applies in the case of registration batches used for Marketing Authorisation/NDA submission, where it is expected the pilot batch size would be no less than 10% of the production scale.

Equipment design and capacity: As discussed in the manufacturing equipment considerations section, it is advisable to use similar process equipment design for scale-up to ensure that the process parameters are transferable to the larger capacity equipment. Ideally, a similar rule to batch size (multiplication scale of 10) would be followed for equipment capacity. The three main considerations are geometric similarity, kinematic similarity, and dynamic similarity (Belwal et al., 2016):

- Geometric similarity requires that all key dimensions in systems of different sizes have the same ratio to each other. Typical key dimensions include vessel diameter, paddle diameter, vessel height, and paddle height from vessel base.
- Kinematic similarity exists when the ratios of the velocities between corresponding points are equal between two systems. Geometric similarities are also evident.
- Dynamic similarities exist between two systems when the ratios of forces between corresponding points are equal. Geometric and kinematic similarities are also evident.

Selection of API: The API used in the scale-up batches should be characterised and its specification should be as close as possible to the API to be used in registration and commercial batches. For the purposes of this comparison, similarity includes synthetic route, site of manufacture, polymorphic form, particle size distribution, purity, and form (hydrates, etc.), as these are often critical material attributes. Changes from here onwards may impact the process, and additional process batches may be required to assess the impact of the change in API. For example, if changing the API synthetic process leads to generation of an additional process impurity, which may not be fully soluble in the vehicle, then this is likely to have a consequential effect on the product's CQAs.

When scaling up the optimised process parameters, careful consideration must be taken of the process(es) involved, the batch size, the duration of the process, and the equipment and its design. Whilst a multiplication factor of 10 is a common default, the actual factor may well be dictated by equipment availability, and therefore adjustments may be required.

7.4 TECHNOLOGY TRANSFER AND VALIDATION

7.4.1 TECHNOLOGY TRANSFER

Technology transfer is a key step in product development and involves an exchange of knowledge between development and manufacturing which can involve both manufacturing process and analytics as outlined in ICH Q10. This knowledge forms the basis for the manufacturing process, control strategy, process validation approach and ongoing continual improvement. The aim is success in larger-scale manufacture, be it non-clinical, clinical, or commercial.

7.4.1.1 Elements of Technology Transfer

Technology transfer involves personnel across a wide range of disciplines including quality assurance and control, project management, formulators and process engineers, and validation scientists. Communication between the sending and the receiving unit should be as early and effective as possible, and the success of the transfer is dependent on all the parties highlighted above, a sound transfer plan/protocol, consistent/controlled procedures, and clear documentation. A detailed assessment of the sending and receiving sites' equipment and environment is required and all parties should agree on the compliance involved and timelines prior to initiation. Prior knowledge is key and information transfer may include:

- Objectives, scope, and responsibilities of sending unit and receiving unit
- Details of instruments used, specifications of raw materials and methods
- Process development report and process flow diagrams
- Experimental design, sampling methods, and acceptance criteria
- Analytical test procedures, product release specifications (e.g., assay and related substances, pH, viscosity, rheology, and sterility), cleaning validation, and method validation report and stability specifications
- Intermediate and raw product stability at different hold points
- Primary and secondary packaging specifications
- Samples and standards provided to the receiving unit as defined in the transfer protocol
- Assisting in feasibility testing before formal transfer

If technology transfer is not performed correctly, it can lead to additional costs, time, and the need to start again if the process and transfer is not fully understood. It can also have an impact on parallel studies (i.e., non-clinical or clinical studies) and certainly will negatively impact the relationship between the two parties. The challenges of managing a Contract Manufacturing Organisation (CMO) relationship are captured by the 5 Cs (Dubois, 2016):

1. *Commitment*: Commitment from both parties to align agreed dates and outcomes, and committing to rapid exchange and response to information.
2. *Cost*: As part of the commitment to the relationship, both parties should agree costs, to allow both to remain competitive and gain a financial return.
3. *Compliance*: Quality issues can certainly affect cost and delivery, but compliance issues can create many more issues, including the health of customers, or in this case, patients.
4. *Capability*: Product and manufacturing technologies must be well-supported and provide differentiators that drive cost, delivery, and margin benefits.

5. *Capacity*: The sponsor assurance that there will be no shut downs, outages, or long lead times that impact schedules. As part of the commitment, it's also important for the Original Equipment Manufacturer (OEM) to plan within the limits of the Contract Manufacturing Organisation's (CMO) capability and capacity.

7.4.1.2 Process Development, QbD, and Robustness

Process robustness is the ability of a process to deliver acceptable drug product quality and performance while tolerating variability in the process and material inputs (Glodek et al., 2006). This may be managed through the choice of manufacturing technology. Eliminating the human element, where possible, reduces the potential for errors. Of course, when considering transfer from development lab to manufacturing, achieving an equivalent process is complicated by scale-up as well as transfer. Something which works on the bench in the laboratory may not necessarily work at the manufacturing site. As such, the scale-up and commercial manufacture should be considered early during the formulation development phase. However, many companies do not wish to outlay on robust technology transfer until much later in the development cycle – for example, Phase III clinical onwards. Unfortunately, the time available decreases and the cost increases the further down the development pathway, and the impact is much greater where a less than robust process is transferred to a commercial plant. Amongst the variables impacted is delay to product launch, issues with regulatory authorities, reduced production rates, increased impact in variation of raw materials, and failed batches.

Quality by Design (Chapter 5) is a set of principles which aim to build quality into the product rather than depending upon end product testing. In practice, it involves taking a systematic approach to product development employing statistical, analytical, and risk-management methodology during the design, development, and manufacturing. With respect to process development, QbD helps to achieve a proper understanding of the manufacturing process which facilitates process validation and any subsequent scale-up and tech transfer. The objective is to identify any CPP and CMA that should be monitored or/and controlled to achieve a product which meets all CQAs.

QbD can also be used to establish a DS, defined as the multidimensional combination and interaction of input variables and process parameters that have been demonstrated to provide assurance of quality. Ultimately, the design space captures the range of CMAs and CPPs which can be tolerated while still achieving the CQAs. Clearly, the tighter the range, the greater the degree of criticality. Such a level of understanding allows the manufacturer to predict where process problems may occur and mitigate against excursions which impact the CQAs. The objectives of pharmaceutical QbD can be summarised as:

- To consistently manufacture a product which meets the CQAs identified in the QTPP. This is achieved by designing a robust process, where changes can be made within the operating range with an assurance of no detrimental effect on the quality of the product.

- To improve process capability and minimise product variability by the means of product and process understanding and appropriate control strategies. Careful design, analysis, and measurement of CPPs (known as Process Analytical Technology [PAT]) can reduce product variability and defects.
- To promote efficiency during product development and manufacturing.
- To enhance root cause analysis and post-approval change management. The goal here is to acquire sufficient understanding of the process such that issues can be easily identified and scale-up or tech transfer activity can be carried out without threat to product quality.

Pharmaceutical Quality by Testing (QbT) ensures the quality of a drug product by implementing and validating a rigid manufacturing process which has evolved through a reactive OFAT approach, and applying a tight release specification to the finished product. The principles set by QbT are not based upon the CMAs and CPPs identified in development, but upon documented observations of previously manufactured batches. Consequently, flexibility for modifications is limited since any change requires submission of a supplement or variation to the relevant competent authority. Figure 7.5 shows the basic differences between QbT and QbD in pharmaceutical development.

7.4.2 PROCESS VALIDATION

Similar to the approach to product development, the now-accepted approach to process validation by the FDA is the process validation lifecycle approach. Although the original FDA guidance for process validation (Guidelines on General Principles of Process Validation, FDA, 1987) did not explicitly state the number of batches required for process validation, three batches had become industry standard. In the case of the EU, a minimum of three validation batches on a commercial scale was expected, but the number of batches could vary based on the variability of the process, the complexity of the process/product, process knowledge gained during development, supportive data at commercial scale during technology transfer and the overall experience of the manufacturer (EMA, 2016).

Updated guidance (Process Validation: General Principles and Practices, 2011), introduced the process validation lifecycle approach, focused on providing assurance that the process was suitably validated using statistical methods. Such an approach may mean that three batches are sufficient, or it may be that more are required to generate the required level of data. The general considerations for process validation are similar to technology transfer and again require an integrated team approach to include skilled personnel across different disciplines (process, analytics, QA, QC, manufacturing, and statistics). Product and process investigations should again be based on sound scientific principles and well-documented with a risk-based approach taken to all attributes (for example, product and quality) and parameters (for example, process and equipment) which will evolve as further information is generated. Validation remain key in providing assurance that a process is sufficiently defined against variability that could impact production, supply, and public health (for example, homogeneity within a batch and consistency across batches).

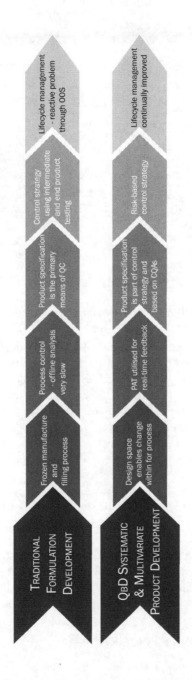

FIGURE 7.5 **(See color insert.)** Comparing traditional pharmaceutical formulation development with a QbD approach. (From ICH, 2009. Q8[R2]: Pharmaceutical development. *ICH Harmonised Tripartite Guideline.*)

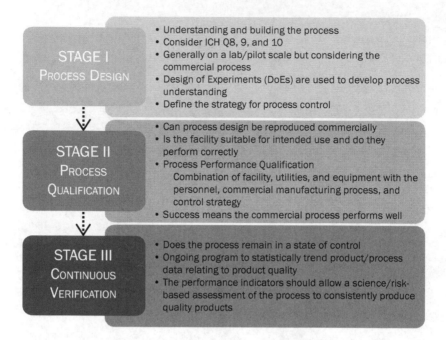

STAGE I
PROCESS DESIGN
- Understanding and building the process
- Consider ICH Q8, 9, and 10
- Generally on a lab/pilot scale but considering the commercial process
- Design of Experiments (DoEs) are used to develop process understanding
- Define the strategy for process control

STAGE II
PROCESS QUALIFICATION
- Can process design be reproduced commercially
- Is the facility suitable for intended use and do they perform correctly
- Process Performance Qualification
  Combination of facility, utilities, and equipment with the personnel, commercial manufacturing process, and control strategy
- Success means the commercial process performs well

STAGE III
CONTINUOUS VERIFICATION
- Does the process remain in a state of control
- Ongoing program to statistically trend product/process data relating to product quality
- The performance indicators should allow a science/risk-based assessment of the process to consistently produce quality products

FIGURE 7.6   (See color insert.) An overview of the process validation lifecycle approach.

Later FDA guidance for process validation (2011) focused on the entire process development approach along with qualification of the process and continuous improvement. For example, the 1987 FDA guidance for Process Validation referred to worst-case conditions; however, in the lifecycle approach such challenging of the system and robustness is performed as part of the process development. The later guidance now states "The commercial manufacturing process and routine procedures must be followed during product performance qualification. The product performance qualification lots should be manufactured under normal conditions by personnel expected to routinely perform each step of each unit operation in the process". An overview of the process validation lifecycle approach is shown in Figure 7.6 and covers three key areas: Process Design (or understanding of the process); Process Qualification (or confirmation of the work performed during the process design); and Continuous Verification (ongoing commercial manufacturing and assurance the product remains the same quality during its lifetime).

Clearly, ensuring product quality both during validation and over the product lifetime is essential when ensuring both safety and efficacy, and this begins during the process design and should be considered even after the product has reached the market.

7.5   COST IMPROVEMENT PROGRAMMES

Cost improvement programmes (CIPs) are usually undertaken once a product is launched in the desired markets and the lifecycle management of the product starts.

These programmes focus on cutting cost of goods (COGs) in a bid to increase the profitability of the marketed product. CIPs are ideal for product that may be granted 180 days exclusivity post-abbreviated new drug application (ANDA) approval, where the benefit of the 180-day period of exclusivity generally outweighs the COGs. However, post the period of exclusivity, COGs become a more important consideration as cheaper generic versions come to market.

All the ingredients used in a pharmaceutical product are manufactured to current good manufacturing practice (cGMP) standards. Due to the quality standards these materials may be sold at a premium, leading to a high COGs, which is one of the major contributors to the cost of product. Although during development, the formulator will take COGs into consideration, the quality of the final product often takes precedence. Post launch, the CIP could be advantageous to a company with strong supply chain management that can negotiate better deals with the material supplier. Alternatively, cheaper suppliers for the same ingredient with same quality material may be sourced and replaced within the product. This is a collaborative effort between supply chain and the formulator and will help reduce the overall costs to the marketed product.

As well as cost of goods, improvements in manufacturing could help reduce the cost of the product; for example, by reducing number of processing steps involved, reducing processing time without compromising quality, incorporating automated processes (such as filling, labelling, checking), or introducing more rigorous contamination controls to prevent batch wastage.

7.6 SUPAC

The FDA guidance for Industry (1997) *Scale-Up* and *Post Approval Changes*: Chemistry, Manufacturing, and Controls; *In Vitro* Release Testing and *In Vivo* Bioequivalence Documentation for Nonsterile Semi-Solid Dosage Forms provides recommendations to pharmaceutical sponsors of new drug applications (NDAs), ANDAs, and abbreviated antibiotic drug applications (AADAs) who intend to change components or composition, manufacturing (process and equipment), scale-up/scale-down of manufacture, and/or site of manufacture of a semi-solid formulation during the post-approval period. The guidance defines the levels of change at three different levels (Levels 1–3). Typically, a Level 1 change is considered as a change unlikely to have an impact on formulation quality and performance, a Level 2 change could have a significant impact on formulation quality and performance, and a Level 3 change is likely to have a significant impact on formulation quality and performance. Also highlighted is the need for chemistry, *in vitro*, and *in vivo* documentation, depending on the level of the change. A summary of the requirements for each change and level of change is provided in Table 7.2. The components and composition focus on changes in excipients in the drug product (changes in preservative are also detailed but not discussed here). Changes to both the manufacturing equipment and process are considered along with the impact of scale-up or down. Finally, changes to the manufacturing site are also included.

TABLE 7.2
SUPAC

Type of Change	Level of Change	Definition	Chemistry Documentation	In vitro Documentation	In vivo Documentation
Components/composition	1	Unlikely to have any detectable impact on formulation quality and performance: Removal of fragrance, flavour, or excipient to impact colour; Change in an excipient up to 5% of approved amount of that excipient; Total additive effect of all excipient changes of 5%; Change in supplier of structure forming excipient (purity ≥ 95%) or technical grade of any other excipient	Updated product release requirement; First production batch long-term stability (annual report)	Not required	Not required
	2	May have significant impact on formulation quality and performance: Change between >5 and ≤10% of individual excipient; Total additive effect of all excipient changes of no more than 10%; Change in supplier/technical grade of structure forming excipient not covered under Level 1; Drug particle size (if suspension)	Updated product release requirement; One batch with three months accelerated data; First production batch long-term stability (annual report)	Release rate of new formulation vs. pre-change formulation (recent lot and comparable age)	Not required

(Continued)

TABLE 7.2 (CONTINUED)
SUPAC

Type of Change	Level of Change	Definition	Chemistry Documentation	In vitro Documentation	In vivo Documentation
	3	Likely significant impact on formulation quality and performance: Any qualitative/quantitative change in excipient above that detailed in Level 2 Change in crystalline form of drug substance (if suspension)	Updated product release requirement One batch with three months accelerated data (or three batches if significant body of data not available) First three production batches long-term stability (annual report)	Release rate of new formulation to be established – because of level of change documentation not required	Full bioequivalence study on the highest strength with in vitro release/other approach for lower strength
Manufacturing equipment	1	Change from nonautomated/nonmechanical equipment to automated or mechanical equipment to transfer ingredients Change to alternative equipment of the same design and principles	Updated product release requirement First production batch long-term stability (annual report)	Not required	Not required
	2	Change in equipment to different design or different operating principles Change in mixing equipment, i.e., low-shear to high shear or vice-versa	Updated product release requirement One batch with three months accelerated data (or three batches if significant body of data not available) First production batch (or three batches if significant body of data not available) long-term stability (annual report)	Release rate of new formulation vs. pre-change formulation (recent lot and comparable age)	Not required
	3	No Level 3 changes expected in this category			

(Continued)

TABLE 7.2 (CONTINUED)
SUPAC

Type of Change	Level of Change	Definition	Chemistry Documentation	*In vitro* Documentation	*In vivo* Documentation
Manufacturing process	1	Changes such as – mixing rate, times, operating speeds, holding times within approved ranges. Order of addition of excipients to either oil or water phase	Application/compendial product release requirements	Not required	Not required
	2	As one but changes outside of approved ranges and any changes in the combining of two phases	Updated product release requirement One batch with three months accelerated data (or three batches if significant body of data not available) First production batch (or three batches if significant body of data not available) long-term stability (annual report)	Release rate of new formulation vs. pre-change formulation (recent lot and comparable age)	Not required
	3	No Level 3 changes expected in this category			
Scale-up/scale-down of manufacture	1	Change in batch size up to and including a factor of 10 times size of pivotal/clinical batch where the same equipment design, SOPs and controls, formulation/ manufacturing procedure are performed under GMP	Updated product release requirement First production batch long-term stability (annual report)	Not required	Not required

(Continued)

TABLE 7.2 (CONTINUED)
SUPAC

Type of Change	Level of Change	Definition	Chemistry Documentation	In vitro Documentation	In vivo Documentation
	2	Change in batch size from beyond a factor of 10 times size of pivotal/clinical batch where the same equipment design, SOPs and controls, formulation/manufacturing procedure are performed under GMP	Updated product release requirement One batch with three months accelerated data First production batch long-term stability (annual report)	Release rate of new formulation vs. pre-change formulation (recent lot and comparable age)	Not required
	3	No Level 3 changes expected in this category			
Site of manufacture	1	Changes consist of site change in single facility with no changes to equipment, SOPs, environmental conditions with personnel common to both manufacturing sites employed and no changes to the BMR occur	Application/compendial product release requirements	Not required	Not required
	2	As 1 but site changes within a contiguous campus or between adjacent city blocks	Updated product release requirement and BMR with facility change First production batch long-term stability (annual report)	Not required	Not required

(Continued)

TABLE 7.2 (CONTINUED)
SUPAC

Type of Change	Level of Change	Definition	Chemistry Documentation	In vitro Documentation	In vivo Documentation
	3	As 1 but site changes to a different campus, i.e., not in contiguous site or adjacent blocks	Updated product release requirement One batch with three months accelerated data (or three batches if significant body of data not available) First production batch (or three batches if significant body of data not available) long-term stability (annual report)	Release rate of new formulation vs. pre-change formulation (recent lot and comparable age)	Not required

7.7   CASE STUDY

As in Chapter 5, the below case study is intended to illustrate some of the principles described throughout this chapter.

CASE STUDY 7.1

AIM

To scale-up and transfer a water-miscible ointment containing a very light sensitive drug for clinical manufacture.

The findings in this case study highlight the importance of:

- Good documentation
- Well-defined process
- The inclusion of formulators/process engineers during technical batch production at the next stage (formulator during process development; process engineer during clinical manufacture)

A water-miscible ointment had been selected through a rigorous program using preformulation and formulation development studies with different *in vitro* tests. A generic process (with light protection) had been implemented for the drug product which involved heating the high molecular weight PEG phase to ensure it was fully molten and subsequent heating of the drug phase containing PEG 400 and a penetration enhancer/solubiliser to the same temperature prior to mixing of the two phases and cooling to ambient temperature. The cooling method was uncontrolled and the batch sizes assessed were ca. 1 Kg.

The information above and details of exact formulation composition were passed to the process engineer. However, because of tight timelines, it was not possible to perform a full QbD process development package (Issue 1). As such, the process above was replicated for a larger batch (10 Kg, which followed the rule of thumb of 1/10 batch size) with no controlled cooling (Issue 2). The viscosity of the larger batches was much lower than the smaller batches and this was considered to be due to the rate of cooling being slower as batch size increases. Furthermore, an increase in a degradation product (attributable to light degradation) was observed. In view of this, some limited process development was performed to explore cooling rate and further protection from light (light filters); a more optimised process was developed before passing the process on to the clinical manufacturing team.

Due to the issues observed during the previous manufacture, it was agreed that a technical batch would be prepared using the clinical manufacturing equipment. The process was transferred and one step during the controlled cooling was to manually manipulate drug product from the side walls of the vessel to ensure that it was not cooling at a faster rate, aiming to avoid a non-homogenous product. It was not clear from the process development work how often the manual manipulation should be performed (Issue 3), only that this should be assessed visually (Issue 4). Due to vacation and the need to progress the technical batch as soon as possible, the process engineer who had worked on the (somewhat limited) process development was not available to be present during the technical batch manufacture (Issue 5). The technical batch was found to contain agglomerates giving it a lumpy consistency. Further process development was performed and bespoke side scrapers to fit on the mixing paddle were manufactured to ensure that there was no build-up of rapidly cooled drug product on the vessel walls.

This case illustrates a number of significant and likely avoidable issues during the development work:

Issue 1 – Process development is a very important part of the development process, and not performing it is a mistake which may actually cost both time and money in the long run.

Issue 2 – A process at a small-scale is not necessarily fully transferable as the scale increases.

Issue 3 – The process documentation transferred between different functions needs to be fully transparent and allow for replication where required.

Issue 4 – Visual assessment under low-light conditions is not the best method quality assurance method and is subjective.

Issue 5 – It is important that the scientists who have knowledge of the product are present at each stage of the manufacture.

BIBLIOGRAPHY

Aulton M.E. (1990). *Pharmaceutical Practice*. Edinburgh: Churchill Livingstone.

Belwal S., et al. (2016). Development and scale up of a chemical process in pharmaceutical industry: a case study. *Int. J. Eng. Res. Appl.* 6 (7) (Part-2): 81–88.

Choy, Y.B. (2011). The rule of five for non-oral routes of drug delivery: Ophthalmic, inhalation and transdermal. *Pharm. Res.* 285: 943–948.

DuBois, B. (2016). The 5 'C's' for CMO Relationships in Pharmaceutical Supply Chain. *21st Century Supply Chain Blog 3 October 2016*. [Online] Available at: http://blog.kinaxis.com/2016/10/5-cs-cmo-relationships-pharmaceutical-supply-chain.

EMA (2001). *Note for Guidance on Process Validation*. CPMP/QWP/848/96, EMEA/CVMP/598/99. London, UK: European Medicines Agency.

EMA (2016). *Guideline on Process Validation for Finished Products – Information and Data to Be Provided in Regulatory Submissions*. EMA/CHMP/CVMP/QWP/BWP/70278/2012-Rev1, Corr.1. London, UK: European Medicines Agency.

Food and Drug Administration (FDA) (1987). *Guideline on General Principles Of Process Validation*.

Food and Drug Administration. (1997). *Guidance for Industry, Scale-Up and Post Approval Changes: Chemistry, Manufacturing, and Controls; In Vitro Release Testing and In Vivo Bioequivalence Documentation for Nonsterile Semi-Solid Dosage Forms*.

Food and Drug Administration. (2011). *FDA Guidance for Industry – Process Validation: General Principles and Practices*.

Gad, S.C. (2008). *Pharmaceutical Manufacturing Handbook, Production and Processes*. Hoboken, NJ: Wiley-Interscience.

Gibson, M. (2004). *Pharmaceutical Preformulation and Formulation*. Boca Raton, FL: HIS Health Group, CRC.

Glodek, M., Liebowitz, S., McCarthy, R., McNally, G., Oksanen, C., Schultz, T., et al. (2006). Process robustness – a PQRI white paper. *Pharm. Eng.* 26: 1–11.

Hu, Y.T., Ting, Y., Hu, J.Y., and Hsieh, S.C. (2017). Techniques and methods to study functional characteristics of emulsion systems. *J. Food Drug Anal.* 25: 16–26. Available at: http://www.nlreg.com/cooling.htm.

ICH (2009). Q8(R2): Pharmaceutical development. *ICH Harmonised Tripartite Guideline*.

ICH (2005). Q9: Quality risk management. *ICH Harmonised Tripartite Guideline*.

ICH (2015). Q10: Pharmaceutical quality development. *ICH Harmonised Tripartite Guideline*.

Maguire, J. and Peng, D. (2015). How to identify critical quality attributes and critical process parameters. *FDA/PQRI 2nd Conference*, October 6, 2015, Bethesda, MD.

Myers, K.J., Reeder, M.F., Bakker, A., and Rigden, M. (1996). Agitating for success. *The Chemical Engineer*. 620: 39–42.

Pandolfe, W.D. (1995). Effect of premix condition, surfactant concentration and oil level on the formation of oil-in-water emulsions by homogenisation. *J. Dispersion Sci. Technol.* 16(7): 633–650.

Ronholt, S., Kirkensgaard, J.J.K., Mortensen, K., and Knudsen, J.C. (2014). Effect of cream cooling rate and water content on butter microstructure during four weeks of storage. *Food Hydrocolloids* 34: 169–176.

Index

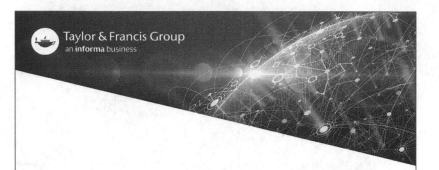